THE HO-HO HOLIEST MEDICINE
Exploring the Power of Divine Laughter

THE HO-HO HOLIEST MEDICINE
Dr. Mitchell J. Bloom, M.D.
Copyright © 2019 by
Laughing Dolphin Press, Greensboro, North Carolina, U.S.A.

THE HO-HO HOLIEST MEDICINE

Exploring the Power of Divine Laughter

Mitchell J. Bloom, MD

A note of caution: I have written this book with the intent of fostering thought, discussion, and laughter. It does not constitute scientific, medical, psychological, emotional, or spiritual advice, nor does this book propose that laughter is always the best medicine, can cure disease, or can solve all the world's problems. I do suggest that laughter be considered as an adjunct to traditional and complementary medical interventions when used under medical supervision and coupled with practical responses when confronted by life's challenges. Readers interested in experimenting with the ideas contained herein should act on them in consultation with a licensed physician, therapist, or other competent professional.

Dr. Mitchell J. Bloom, M.D

About Dr. Mitchell J. Bloom

Dr. Bloom is a board-certified Medical Doctor and board-certified hypnotist who combines Traditional Medicine with Affordable Cell Therapy. The Regenerative Medicine Treatments he uses - can be used for most painful orthopedic conditions, are completely non-surgical, have an 80-90% success rate according to published studies and are a fraction of the cost of Stem Cell Therapy.

For the past thirty-plus years, Dr. Bloom has also been on a journey of unraveling the human mind to explore the underlying reasons for why certain challenging people, situations and medical conditions appear in our lives. In this process, he made a revolutionary discovery with profound implications.

A byproduct of this discovery is a treatment Dr. Bloom developed called "LaughGnosis™." LaughGnosis is a technique that combines laughter with hypnosis to achieve "Gnosis." Gnosis is knowledge into humanity's true Divine nature which, according to some spiritual teachings, comes from knowing oneself at the deepest level, and is how to know "God." LaughGnosis, which is described in this book, is a treatment Dr. Bloom uses to treat real physical diseases and psychological conditions arising from repressed emotional causes.

Dr. Bloom is a doctor that patients with physical and emotional pain turn to, especially when all else fails. For more information about Dr. Bloom, and for workshops or Skype sessions based on this book, please visit www.HoHoHoly.com or www.AffordableCells.com.

Table of Contents

Glossary.. 10

Preface... 18

Chapter One: STOP: Don't Buy This Book 19

Chapter Two: No Place to Hide.. 21

Chapter Three: Turning Pain into Bliss with Laughter 25

    Stopping: The Power to "Gain Wait" 27

    No Thoughts, No Pain 32

    God—The Misunderstood Comedian...................................... 36

Chapter Four: The Paradigm Shift 39

    Understanding Miracles 39

    Miracles Greater Than These... 40

Chapter Five: The Science and Religion of Miracles............... 43

    The Joke of "Reality" According to Nobel Laureates and Scholars...... 44

    Laughter – The Natural Response to a Reality That's Not Real............ 50

    Reality According to Religion, Philosophy and Sacred Scriptures 52

    The Illusory World.. 54

    No Time, No Space – Just Laughter 56

Chapter Six: The Miracle of Laughter..................................... 58

    Inspiration for the Cover of This Book.................................... 59

    Laughing at the Illusion of Hell 61

    Laughing Like Our Lives Depend On It................................... 62

    Laughter, The Detergent to Clean Away Suffering.................. 64

    Laughing at Everything... 66

    The Sweet 16 Reasons to Laugh at Our Conditioned Thoughts........... 68

    Accessing "The Zone" to Experience Miracles......................... 71

Chapter Seven: The Inconvenient Joke.................................... 73

Dr. Bloom's Allegory – A New Model of Reality......................76

The Easiest Way to End Wars, Terrorist and School Shootings 80

The Greatest Magic Show on Earth 84

Laughing Too Hard: Oops—The Disappearance of the Universe........85

Laughing Away Old Memories 86

Why The Inconvenient Joke is so Inconvenient 93

How to Live as "Spiritual Beings Having a Human Experience"..........95

Laughter: The Rational Response to a Reality That's Not Real............96

Chapter Eight: Dissolving Negative Emotions...................... 98

How to Worry Effectively 102

Changing Our Ideas about What Requires Change.............103

Chapter Nine: Weapons of Mass Distraction..........................106

The Greatest Terrorist That Ever Lived is Closer than You Think.....107

Chapter Ten: Thought Addicts Anonymous..........................110

The Deadliest Vice of All 112

Chapter Eleven: The "F" Word 114

The Benefit of "F"ing Someone 115

Ten Steps to Forgiveness.................................117

Chapter Twelve: Unconditional Love Meets Adolph Hitler 119

What is Love?.................................121

Embarrassing Confessions.................................123

The Upside-Down Universe.................................125

Chapter Thirteen: Entering The Zone at the Speed of Laughter 127

Redefine and Shine 130

Ho-Ho-Holy Communication 131

The Joke Embedded in the Emotional Scale.................132

Chapter Fourteen: The Hero's Journey 134

Embracing The Great Abyss.................................137

Bypassing The Hero's Journey.................................141

Beliefs that Interfere with This Laughter.................142

Chapter Fifteen: Is Laughter the Best Medicine?.................144

The Psychology of Disease.................................146

The Psychology of Health..148

The Inconvenient Dogma of Biology...149

Treating Root Causes of Disease for the Best Results...........152

Chapter Sixteen: Miracles..**154**

Miracles in Disguise...156

Modifying Genetic Diseases...158

Irony Deficiency/God's Humor 101 160

Experiencing Miracles 164

Greater Miracles than Jesus...167

Wake up Laughing from "Death"...169

Chapter Seventeen: Dying to Wake Up **172**

Prisoners of Our Own Mind...174

Laughing Our Way Home..176

Laughing at Death 177

Unleashing the Wizard Within...179

The Inspiration Gained from Expiration.................................181

Chapter Eighteen: Finding Heaven on Earth **187**

Trading Heaven for Knowledge...189

No Thanks! Trading Knowledge Back for Heaven 191

Chapter Nineteen Changing Faults into Laughter **193**

Living in The Zone in Our Daily Life..195

Smiling: A Way of Preventing "Truth Decay".......................198

Chapter Twenty: Understanding God's Jokes— The Sherlock Holmes

Approach **202**

The "Sybil War" Inside Our Mind..204

God's Misunderstood Jokes...205

Shining the Light on Shadows..207

Amazed by the Maze..208

Questioning God's Ethics..209

Laughing Our Way Out of the Illusion.....................................210

Becoming an Alchemist of Our Life..211

Chapter Twenty-One: The Fifth Noble Truth **214**

Chapter Twenty-Two: Laughterism, The Ho-Ho-Holiest Religion 218

Laughter, The Language of God...220

Seven Advantages 222

Chapter Twenty-Three: LaughGnosis™, the Ha-Ha-Happiest Path to God...224

What is LaughGnosis? 226

More benefits of LaughGnosis 229

Christian Views of Hypnosis...233

Chapter Twenty-Four: Laughing Our Way to Heaven 236

Waking Up from The American Nightmare.............................237

Global Chaos: The Punchline with a Mighty Punch.................239

Delivering the Knockout Punchline 241

Bursting the Spiritual Bubble...243

Global Evolution through Laughter 245

Saying Goodbye to The Illusory World...................................249

Being the First to Laugh 252

References..255

NOTE: All words may have baggage, especially words like Jesus, God, and ego. To set the stage and get the most benefit from this book, I recommend that you let go of other associations you may have with the following words and names, and temporarily use the definitions in this book.

Glossary

Adam and Eve: Two biblical figures who can also represent the origin of Dualistic thinking (see dualistic) and false knowledge.

Awakening: The process of enlightenment – waking up from the "Illusory World" (see "*Illusory World*").

Cosmic Joke: The Joke we play on ourselves by forgetting to laugh at the ironies that arise from believing we are victims of a cruel world, despite Nobel Laureate quantum physicists describing the world as essentially an illusory Hall of Mirrors that merely reflects back what is in front of it.

This book explores this seemingly Inconvenient Joke in great detail. (I use the terms "Cosmic Joke, Inconvenient Joke, God's Joke and Powerful Joke" interchangeably.) Although this "Joke" can often sometimes seem overwhelmingly cruel, this book invites you to see if it is possible to laugh at all the ironies that may arise from refusing to laugh. This book suggests that this laughter may enable us to see "God" as a "Misunderstood Comedian," and that laughing at Her Jokes can help us to laugh our way out of our world of suffering - and into "God's" Empowering World of Heaven on Earth.

The Cosmic Joke is better to be laughed at than described. It is not something that can be defined in a few paragraphs or a few chapters. It should be understood <u>by the time you finished this book</u> and laughed at as you go through your life.

Dr. Bloom's Allegory: Based on quantum physics, this allegory explains how, despite all our diligent ongoing efforts, we often fail to achieve true, long-lasting peace and happiness, and how this goal can be achieved through Powerful Laughter at the Cosmic Joke. For a full description, please see Chapter 7.

Disempowered Resistance: The illusion of disempowerment is based on the belief that we are innocent victims of a cruel world – victims justified in our anger, fears, and resistance. "Disempowered" resistance is transformed through Powerful Laughter into "this-empowered" strength.

Divine Laughter: Laughter at the Cosmic Joke (see Cosmic Joke).

Dualistic/Duality: Divided into individual parts. This belief contradicts physics assertions that view ultimate reality as one undivided, non-local, perfectly interconnected Whole. Dualism sets the stage for the dichotomy of "I" and "other." Believing there is someone outside of us sets the stage for fear, jealousy, and anger, which predispose to competition and conflict.

Ego: The part of our mind that appears to help us navigate the Illusory World (see "*Illusory World*"). This Illusory World consists of a world and conditioned thought system which the ego itself created. Our conditioned thoughts create the belief that who we are is defined by our beliefs, emotions, and memories. These thoughts also create the illusion of separation from our Interconnected Wholeness with All That Is. This book proposes that laughing at our conditioned thoughts helps us transcend our sense of separation, our ego, and the Illusory World it created, so that we may live in a Heaven on Earth.

Empowered Peace: The state in which there is a clear mind without any distracting or disempowering thoughts or beliefs of "victimization," and an openness to creative ideas and epiphanies. It is the functional state of people living in "The Zone."

Enlightenment: Our natural state of oneness with everyone and everything, including with God. It is knowing Who We Really Are, beyond our body, thoughts, stories and our roles in society. Enlightenment is recognizing that same Divine Essence within everything in existence that seems so deeply hidden, but yet so obvious once we stop seeking and start laughing.

Equanimity/Being Equanimous: An equilibrium of mind in which everything is observed without any craving for things to be different. By seeing every event and sensation as neutral, equanimous people are more fully present and live in "The Zone."

Frankenstein Monster: Any person or situation that challenges us – a debilitating or life-threatening disease, chronic pain, a verbally or physically abusive spouse, a demanding boss, the IRS, the Global Elite, a corrupt politician, the loss of a job, or any memory or any limiting belief that prevents us from experiencing Who We Really Are (see "Know Thyself").

Glossary: A list defining unusual words and expressions used in the text. **Caution**: If this list or anything else is taken too seriously, it may cause excessive thinking instead of the primary objective of mind activity – to remind us to laugh at our thoughts and at the Inconvenient Joke and enable us to laugh ourselves into Heaven on Earth.

Gnosis: Knowledge into humanity's true Divine nature which, according to some spiritual teachings, comes from knowing oneself at the deepest level, and is how to know God.

Gnostic State: An altered state of consciousness in which a person's mind is perfectly focused on one single point, thought, or goal. The gnostic state is used to bypass the "filters" of the conscious mind and is necessary for working with many forms of magic as well as with hypnosis.

God: The Core Divine Essence within everyone and everything in existence that is always connected and ever-present.

God is well beyond words and is best defined as being undefined. Any words we use to describe God misdirect us to the mind's version of God. The authentic experience of God, however, does not exist within the mind.

We experience God when we laugh away our thoughts about God and everything else. Since the harder we try to define God the further we get from the experience of God, let's go on to the next definition.

God's Joke: Please see "The Cosmic Joke" and "The Inconvenient Joke," as they are used interchangeably with "God's Joke."

Hall of Mirrors: The belief supported by several Nobel Laureates that the world is essentially an illusory Hall of Mirrors that reflect back what is in front of it.

Illusion of Hell: When the world we see causes us to experience a form of Hell – living in an evil, cruel, and dangerous world, full of chaos and suffering. (This book proposes that laughing at God's Jokes can help us break out of this Illusion of Hell.)

Illusory World: According to a growing number of quantum physicists our experience of reality is essentially an illusion; a holographic Hall of Mirrors created by our thoughts.

A Course in Miracles, which is the bible of spirituality and metaphysics for many people, says, "Into eternity, where all is one, there crept a tiny, mad idea, at which the Son of God remembered not to laugh." In our for-getting to laugh, we took this "tiny mad idea" seriously, and it became our reality.

In other words, we were in "The Zone," having a Heavenly experience of our Oneness with God, when we wondered what it would be like to be-lieve the holographic Hall of Mirrors is real and experience living outside of Heaven. We remembered not to laugh at that idea, became mesmerized by the idea, created a dream-like illusion we call reality based on the idea and believe that this "Illusory World" is all that exists of reality.

Since we got sucked into The Illusion by not laughing, this book proposes that our return to Heaven may be achieved by remembering to laugh at our "Illusory World"... what we call our world.

The Inconvenient Joke: The Cosmic Joke (see "Cosmic Joke") that, once fully understood and wholeheartedly laughed at, will enable us to no longer suffer. Laughing at This Joke allows us to let go of cravings, aver-sions, and feelings of lack or limitation. This Powerful Laughter empowers us to align with the miracles of God. Nevertheless, it can be highly incon-venient as can any personal or cultural shift of consciousness and world view.

Jesus: The real or metaphorical being who was perfectly aligned with God. Jesus brought us transformational teachings that can best be learned once we let go of negative associations that some have placed on His name.

Karma: The principle of cause and effect where intent and actions of an individual (cause) influence the future of that individual (effect). It is based on Newton's 3rd law: "For every action, there is an equal and oppo-site reaction." Whatever pattern of energy we produce will ultimately come back to us to equalize the effect.

Know Thyself: The core of many spiritual practices. This knowing goes deeper than any superficial knowledge of Who We Really Are or the face we show to the world. Mohammed said, "He who knows his own self, knows God." Since we are created in God's image, to know ourselves can help us know God.

The Light of God: This Light represents God. It is the Source of all miracles and the love and peace that goes beyond understanding. It is the source of Heaven on Earth. Being in "The Zone" is the way to align ourselves with this Light.

LaughGnosis™: The combining of Powerful Laughter with hypnosis in order to achieve Gnosis (please see "Gnosis").

Miracle: A wonderful event that is in some way contrary to our expectations and appears to be unexplainable.

Nirvana: A condition of great peace and bliss through the extinction of all desires and passions, created by absorption into the experience of Oneness with God.

Non-Dualistic: The awareness that everything is "One perfectly united Whole." This refers to the state of consciousness described in spiritual teachings and by a growing number of physicists in which everything is non-local and interconnected. Even though we may appear to be separate and disconnected due to our seemingly separate bodies, at the deepest level of our Being, we are all interconnected in a non-dualistic way. Seeing "others" as perfectly united with "us" sets the stage for cooperation, admiration, trust, and Unconditional Love.

Powerful Joke: The Cosmic Joke that empowers us to Wake Up to Who We Really Are (See "Cosmic Joke" and "Who We Really Are").

Powerful Laughter: The empowering Laughter that is experienced when we Laugh at the Cosmic Joke.

Pronouns: All pronouns in this book should be read as though they have quotations around them. Although within our interconnected, non-local, non-dualistic reality, there is no such thing as "you," "us," "them," "she," "he," etc., for convenience and by convention, traditional pronouns are used without quotation marks.

Resisting What Is: Being out of alignment with people or situations through a lack of Equanimity and Disempowered Resistance (see "Equanimity" and "Disempowered Resistance"). Resistance creates negative emotions, more sin, and distortions on one's lens (see "Dr. Bloom's Allegory" and "Sin").

Sin: Being out of alignment with the Light of God and believing in the illusion of separation from Who We Really Are (also see Enlightenment).

Test-tickles: The negative emotions that arise from our Frankenstein Monsters. They serve as a test to make sure we are laughing at the Cosmic Joke. When we are taking the world too seriously and have taken a bit of a snooze from laughing at The Joke, these test-tickles serve as our tickle-alarm.

True Self: The reflection of us that is most aligned with the Light of God.

Victimizers: Health challenges, people, situations, thoughts, beliefs, or memories that were cosmically designed as the rocket fuel necessary to push our buttons and motivate us to Awaken to Who We Really Are. These perceived Frankenstein Monsters are our greatest teachers of forgiveness and unconditional love. They guard the doorway to the miracles that lie within each of us.

Vipassana: The practice of continued close attention to thoughts and sensations through which we ultimately see the true nature of existence. It is often done as a ten-day, eleven hours per day course in which we are encouraged not to move during meditation and to observe noble silence throughout (silence of body, speech, and mind).

Waking Up: The process of becoming enlightened.

Wake Up Laughing: The process of consciously Laughing at our thoughts and at the Cosmic Joke to wake up from the "Illusory World" (see "Illusory World").

Who We Really Are: The essence of everyone and everything in existence that is not affected by any thoughts or bodily conditions. It is the part of us that doesn't change, never dies, and is connected with everyone and everything (see "Know Thyself").

X-ray glasses: The imaginary glasses we can use to see God's humor wherever we go (they are necessary to wake up laughing).

The Zone: The place where passion, excitement, and determination meet equanimity. When we are in "The Zone" we're in a state of intense single-minded and absolute immersion in the present moment. We are so utterly absorbed in an activity that the activity itself is intrinsically rewarding, and other needs become negligible. It is the ultimate state of harnessing our emotions, and we experience it as pure, focused motivation. This motivation is then positively energized and aligned with the activity, resulting in a timeless state of flow – the state in which there is no trying. There is only effortless movement, without thinking. It is always accompanied by a spontaneous feeling of absolute bliss. There is the complete loss of a separate self and the subjective experience of time. From this very powerful state, miraculous things may happen.

Preface

I would like to thank all the Late-Night Comedians who helped inspire me to take in all the toxic garbage of this chaotic world and turn it into brilliant rainbows that bring us laughter and joy.

I would especially like to thank you, the reader, for having the curiosity to explore the possibility of helping in the evolution of consciousness so that we may live in a joyful, harmonious and loving world through Powerful Laughter.

I would also like to thank everyone else, including all our saintly teachers, Nobel Laureate Physicists, and all the infuriating spouses, obnoxious bosses, and megalomaniacal politicians of the world.

Thank you all for taking part in this seemingly tumultuous and often horrifying dance of consciousness and for driving me to ask those burning questions that kept me awake many nights, staring at my ceiling:

- What on Earth is going on here? (this is the extremely sanitized version of my question).
- Is "God" vindictive and cruel, or could He be a Misunderstood Comedian?
- If God is a Comedian, can my patients live more empowered, happier, healthier and longer lives by understanding His sense of humor?

"Nothing kills the ego like playfulness, like laughter. When you start taking life as fun, the ego has to die, it cannot exist anymore."
— Osho

Chapter One
STOP: Don't Buy This Book

I went to a bookstore one day and found an excellent self-help book. Since it looked like the perfect book, I decided to buy it. Then, out of the blue, I heard a voice say, "STOP." When I turned around, there was nobody there, so I proceeded to the checkout, where the voice said in an even louder voice, "STOP. Don't buy this book." I looked around again and saw no one, and thought to myself, uh oh, they put people away for things like this!

I felt compelled to bargain with the voice, promising this would be the last self-help book I bought. After all, once I finished reading this excellent book, I should be in an enlightened state and not need to buy any more books. Again, the voice said, "STOP!"

I stopped to think. I had spent most of my life in pursuit of happiness, believing all the answers would be found in the next self-help book. What if the answers are beyond books and even beyond thoughts? "What if laughter is the answer?"

What if Mark Twain was right? What if: "The human race has one really effective weapon, and that is laughter"?

What if Powerful Laughter enabled me to see the most challenging people and situations in my life - my "Frankenstein Monsters," from a light-hearted yet powerful perspective? What if it gave me the ability to live in "The Zone" and enjoy a longer and better quality of life, better health and more of a feeling of empowerment?

This book provides you with an invitation to see if it is possible to look at your world from a perspective supported by Nobel Prize Laureates, the core of major religions, and metaphysical teachings. Using this fact-based perspective as much as possible, this book invites you to see if it is possible to laugh at your Frankenstein Monsters in order to live your life in "The Zone," to access your True Power.

To maximize the potential transformational power of this book, I encourage you to consider who your greatest Frankenstein Monsters are, and keep them in mind as you read.

Before you read this book, I also encourage you to skim the *Glossary.* Words like "God," "Jesus" and "ego" all have associated baggage. To get the most benefit from this book, I recommend referring to the glossary definition. To make reading of the glossary easier, the first time these terms are used, they will be in ***bold, italic and underlined.*** Glossary terms like The Divine Laughter, The Cosmic Joke, The Inconvenient Joke, etc. may not be clear until after you have finished reading this book.

But before you read this book, I want to warn you. This book is not for those who wish to continue believing they are victims and insist on taking life very seriously. Also, this book is based on a near-death experience I had, and based on my interpretation of information and not intended as professional advice. As you know, you are completely free to accept or reject as much as you like. All I know is when I live my life as though this book is true, I am much more joyful and peaceful and live in "The Zone" much more.

I would also like to warn you that I am not enlightened and that this book is not for everyone. If you are a serious seeker in search of vital spiritual information that will bring you supreme enlightenment, perfect health, or power over others, you will not find it in this book. But if you would like to have a few giggles about "oh so serious" topics, I suggest you put away your serious mind and come with me on a journey into the heart of the most Earth-shattering Joke ever told. Let's go on a journey of reclaiming our ability to laugh at this oh so serious world.

But before we go, I have something to confess. I am not a comedian. If you would like funny jokes to make you happy, don't buy this book. But if you would like to access ***Powerful Laughter*** that can help you take back your power to change your world in a way that is the best for all concerned, I invite you to join me to explore the Ho-Ho-Holiest Medicine.

"Beneath this entire universe is the Cosmic Joke, and tapping into that level of the game is almost like going beyond enlightenment. You're tapping into the very bliss of God, applauding His intricate set-ups, and of course, rolling in the aisles at the magnificent punch line."
— Sharon Janis, *Spirituality for Dummies*

Chapter Two
No Place to Hide

Although I had been a medical doctor and a spiritual seeker for over thirty years, I felt no closer to **enlightenment** than when my spiritual path began. I'd read stacks of the latest spiritual books and attended countless workshops, but these had only filled my mind with interesting party conversation that seemed to sometimes impress my friends and feed my **ego.**

Instead of bringing lightheartedness, my "spirituality" caused me to be very judgmental. Although I tried to use spirituality to make me happy, it was making me quite miserable.

Life seemed to be full of ironies. I went to medical school to help people. Before starting medical school, I had no idea that medications would be a leading cause of death. Although drugs and surgeries are sometimes beneficial and absolutely necessary, after completing medical school, I felt devastated when some of my patients died due to the side effects of medications.

I spent many sleepless nights staring at the ceiling, feeling confused about the medical system. All those grueling years of medical school and residency seemed wasted. I wondered what I had done with my life and whether there was a safe and effective alternative to medications and surgeries.

During this same time, I was feeling intense anger toward several world leaders. This anger was so deep, I felt like my blood would boil whenever I saw them on TV.

In addition to anger, I experienced a great deal of fear. Among many other fears, I had an enormous fear of being killed by terrorism. It was frustrating to realize that everything I did to ensure my safety never seemed like it would be enough.

After the 2001 terrorist attacks in New York City, Washington D.C, and Connecticut, I reviewed evacuation procedures wherever I was, in case of another attack. I always tried to have a full tank of gas and kept my running shoes next to the door.

When I heard the Department of Homeland Security advising Americans to buy duct tape to prepare for potential chemical and biological warfare, I quickly left the house to get duct tape.

I went to two stores, but both were out of duct tape. Panic struck... What if the terrorists had hijacked the duct tape delivery trucks? What if there was a national duct tape shortage? What if all the duct tape manufacturers were kidnapped by terrorists? Maybe I could help more people if I gave up my medical practice and became a duct tape manufacturer!

The third store had four rolls of Scotch tape. I bought them, though still frantically seeking duct tape before the terrorists attacked. I finally found one roll of duct tape, and with a sigh of relief, bought it. I quickly drove home, feeling a bit like a burglar in his getaway car with the stash.

As I began applying the duct tape around each window, a fresh wave of panic overwhelmed me when I realized that I didn't have enough tape to seal them all – let alone deal with the fireplace.

Imagining radioactivity pouring into my home, I wanted to run away to find a place of safety but didn't know where that might be. Realizing this idea was irrational, I noticed how the desire to run away seemed to be a repeating pattern for me. I had run away from challenging people and situations and had engaged in many forms of escapism my entire life, only to find similar challenges no matter what I did or how far I ran. If I had a nickname, it would have been Dr. Skedaddle.

This skedaddling impulse became so intense about the political situation in the U.S.A., I gave up the American Dream of having everything I ever wanted, to move to New Zealand where I faced worse problems. This intense inner turmoil inspired me to write this book. Writing this book helped me realize that **the more diligently I searched for inner peace and safety, the more difficult it was to find.** Focusing on my sense of vulnerability created more fearful thoughts, which only created a greater feeling of vulnerability. Although I thought anger and fear were motivating me to do what was necessary to feel more peaceful and safer, they caused me to feel more at risk and angry.

In my Pain Medicine practice, I saw numerous patients who had seen multiple other physicians and practitioners and had gone through virtually every treatment known to man, yet continued to experience pain. In working to unravel their condition, I found the physical pain was often preceded or complicated by emotional pain and did not always respond as well to my Regenerative/Cell Based Treatments. This emotional pain was often the result of an abusive spouse, demanding boss, the IRS, corrupt politicians, global chaos, the loss of a job, or any other form of "**_Franken-stein Monster._**" Whether escaping through alcohol, sex, overeating, being a workaholic, drugs, or even spirituality, they all seemed to have their unique method of skedaddling.

While feeling like part of a collective punching bag and surrendering to the possibility of never finding peace, I spontaneously began to laugh at the possibility of "God" being a Comedian playing an Inconvenient **_Cosmic Joke_** on us. It seemed as though He was wondering how long it would take before we realized that even if we flew to Pluto, it wouldn't be far enough, because the challenges from which we were trying to escape were coming from our own mind.

This laughter – **not at the challenging people or events, but at our thoughts about them** – was such a relief. It was the alchemy that helped me see the intense agony of our pitiful existence from a place of peace, clarity and, paradoxically, a feeling of empowerment. This clarity helped me realize that I needed to return to the U.S.A. to laugh at my intense fears – those same fears that drove me halfway around the world to avoid. This forced me to surrender to God's sense of humor, to help access this Ho-Ho-Holy Medicine.

I would like to share this Ho-Ho-Holy Medicine with you, so perhaps you too can gain more comfort, inner peace, and a feeling of empowerment by laughing at His funny, yet extremely challenging Jokes.

"If a person can laugh totally, wholeheartedly, not holding anything back at all, in that very moment something tremendous can happen because laughter, when it is total, is absolutely egoless, and that is the only condition in which to know God, to be egoless."
— Osho

Chapter Three
Turning Pain into Bliss with Laughter

As a Medical Doctor specializing in the treatment of pain for the past 30 years, I achieved the most dramatic longest-lasting results when correcting the root causes of the pain by using modalities I learned in medical school, at Integrative Medicine conferences, and by reading Medical literature. I never considered the possibility of finding a more profound and more transformational root cause of pain by doing a 10-day **_Vipassana_** meditation - one that not only eliminated my pain but turned it into such intense Bliss, it was beyond any type of Bliss I ever imagined possible.

I became especially aware of my pain during the first day of the ten-day meditation course. I had been sitting in noble silence – not moving for eleven hours – and developed excruciating pain in my buttocks. Every time I sat on my cushion, I entered a time warp of intense pain that made each second seem like hours, and each minute seem like days.

Not only did the meditation leaders expect us to sit in silence, but to sit perfectly still. When I looked around, it seemed as though everyone in the meditation hall was sitting effortlessly, like perfect statues of Buddha. I felt I was the only person squirming on my cushion and writhing in excruciating agony, wondering if the timekeeper had taken a snooze.

I kept thinking about how I could be on a beach in the Bahamas sipping a Piña Colada. Instead, I was sitting in a meditation hall in absolute misery, seeking enlightenment. How enlightened is that?

To top it off, I was a medical doctor with expertise in pain management who had spent most of my life learning how to alleviate pain. Yet there I was, intentionally creating it.

Not only did I experience excruciating pain in my butt, but I also had great difficulty maintaining noble silence. How could I be expected to maintain complete silence when I had eaten Mexican food for lunch?

I must admit, I did break my silence that day. I felt very guilty about it until finding out that silence means no verbalization......from the mouth.

I considered how yogis required years of meditation before performing **miracles**, while I was able to perform a miracle in a matter of moments - by turning a soft meditation cushion into solid stone the moment I sat on it.

I was completely convinced I would eventually find the perfect number and configuration of pillows to allow me to feel comfortable. Several days later, I realized that this belief was highly delusional.

It boggled my mind how a pile of plush, soft, velvety cushions in one moment could turn into a torture gadget from Hell, even if I stacked the cushions the height of Mount Everest.

What began as a desire for Self-Realization had turned into an experience of Self-Mutilation. The only Self-Realization I had was the realization that I was a complete jerk – intentionally spending my vacation in some kind of spiritual concentration camp from Hell, practicing a Buddhist version of S&M.

I grumbled to myself, wondering if our meditation guide was trained at a special Buddhist Center in Guantanamo Bay by a descendant of Adolf Hitler, and whether tomorrow's session would begin with a waterboarding meditation.

Sitting in agony for eleven hours a day once again triggered my deep-seated craving to run away from discomforts in my never-ending pursuit of happiness. I was convinced that happiness was always just around the corner, and that I could always find it later once I ran away from wherever I was now.

My compulsion to run, which had always run my life, was now running me into a mind-created Hell of my own making. Once I stopped running and had a relatively quiet mind, everything I had run away from all these years came running into my mind, and seemed to be conspiring to show me who was the boss.

It seemed as though my pain was my lion and my mind was the lion tamer. I was intentionally locking myself in a lion's den and throwing away the key. All I had to tame this ferocious lion was my mind.

Any craving for comfort intensified the pain and caused the lion to become more ferocious. The more I resisted the lion by squirming on my cushion or by having any negative thoughts about the pain, the more ferocious it became.

It soon became clear that my mind was my most ferocious lion of all; my mind was generating the resistance that intensified the pain. So, I was trying to use my mind to tame my mind, which seemed as likely to succeed as a self-taming lion.

Stopping: The Power to "Gain Wait"

As I spiraled down into the depths of this cycle of defeat, I suddenly became aware of what I was doing to myself yet again by wanting to run away. This time, I saw that the same compulsion to run that I thought had been keeping me safe all these years ironically seemed to be the very compulsion that was fueling my crazed suffering.

That's when it hit me. What if, instead of running, I just STOPPED and completely accepted my pain as it was? What if my biggest problem was a WAIT problem? All those years I believed I needed to not just sit there but to do something. Maybe now was the time to learn how to not only do something, but sit there.......and "gain WAIT."

The more I was able to stop my resistance and experience the pain as pure sensation, the less intense the pain became. As long as I had no cravings for comfort and no aversion to the discomfort, the lion was tame. This happened when my mind was in perfect equilibrium, without any internal story about the sensations I was experiencing. In this state of **_Equanimity_,** the pain was experienced as pure sensation.

27

Despite this realization, my compulsion to run became more intense by the moment. As this compulsion intensified, so did the pain. As the pain intensified, so did the compulsion to run. It was a vicious cycle that made me feel like an absolute failure, utterly defeated by my craving to be spiritual.

My pain was teaching me that if responding to my aversion and craving to leave was the cause of my suffering, maybe stopping and facing everything completely from a place of Equanimity could be the cure. Perhaps, through this process of patience and surrender, I could achieve my ideal wait.

I felt fortunate that my type of pain was perfect for this purpose – the extreme discomfort resolved within a few minutes of rising from the meditation cushions and wasn't doing long-term physical damage. I believe that most pain is present for a reason, even if it is simply to get us to a doctor who can treat its root cause with the safest and most effective treatment or, failing a complete cure, to teach us to rise above the fear, anxiety, and anger that can come with chronic pain.

These realizations helped me realize that my greatest challenges can also be my greatest teachers.

Empowered Peace vs. Disempowered Resistance

I realized that my fear and desire to run away caused me to feel disempowered. I had felt entirely justified in my anger, fears, and resistance. I felt like a poor innocent victim of a corrupt and cruel world. I had always believed in resisting evil people with force and using anger to drive me to action. But this anger and resistance toward the cruel world seemed to be creating a feeling of "Disempowered Resistance."

This "Disempowered Resistance" caused me to respond in ineffectual ways. My resistance turned out to be highly effective... for my "*Victimizers.*"

I began to see that these "Victimizers" – health challenges, people, situations, thoughts, and painful memories – were Cosmically designed as the rocket fuel necessary to push my buttons. Their goal was to motivate me to be as effective as possible in the face of adversity, to learn to function in "*The Zone.*"

Instead, my fear and anger seemed to be empowering my "Victimizers" while disempowering me. The anxiety caused by these empowered Victimizers resulted in negative beliefs that worsened the underlying condition, creating even more fear and anger. This whirlwind of agitation had prevented me from opening my mind to creative solutions.

Throughout my career, I've seen patients who had "Victimizers" in their lives. For many of them, these challenges occurred just prior to the onset of, and seemed to precipitate, their health conditions. There was often a person or situation that challenged them – a verbally or physically abusive spouse, a demanding boss, an IRS audit, an economic collapse, or the loss of a job. Wouldn't it be nice if we could use such challenges as the rocket fuel necessary to grow, evolve, and function in "The Zone"?

I had always been fascinated by The Zone. Elite athletes accomplished miraculous feats by being in The Zone. People who function in The Zone describe it as a place of intense and equanimous single-minded immersion in the present moment. It is the ultimate state of harnessing one's emotions in the performance of an activity. The Zone is "skill in action," an absolute focused motivation that is positively energized and aligned with the activity. It is a timeless and complete state of flow, a state in which there is no trying, only effortless movement, without thinking. There is such absolute absorption in the activity that the activity itself is intrinsically rewarding, while other needs become negligible, just as someone entirely absorbed in a creative task may forget the time or need to eat or sleep. In The Zone, there is the complete loss of a sense of separate self, and the subjective experience of time is altered. From this very powerful state, miraculous things can happen.

People functioning in The Zone feel empowered and full of excitement, passion, determination, and absolute focus, balanced with Deep Inner Peace and equanimity in a state of "Empowered Peace." They have a clear mind, free of any distracting or disempowering thoughts or beliefs.

I decided to try out these exciting ideas with my intense pain as the hours of sitting went on, using it as the rocket fuel to help me access The Zone.

For the next few meditation sessions, I focused on projecting my pain to different parts of the room and out the window. This turned out to be a very successful way to eradicate the pain.

Although my pain was completely gone after this little exercise, this process seemed too easy. What if the pain had a greater lesson?

During the following sessions, I dissociated myself from the pain by watching myself from the ceiling. This also successfully eradicated the pain. Though the pain was gone entirely, this also seemed too easy. I felt as though the pain had a still more significant lesson, so I associated back into the pain and continued this fascinating exploration.

On the fourth day of meditation, I realized that I was still caught in the same pattern of running away, this time from the pain. I was either over here projecting the pain over there, or I was over there, watching the pain over here. I was still in that same pattern of trying to escape from my painful reality, treating my pain and the painful people, situations, and health conditions in my life as Victimizers that were out to get me.

Over the next few days, I worked on healing this sense of victimization by seeing no separation between me and the pain. Eventually, I felt as though I had "merged" with it. When I did, the pain took on an entirely new quality, in which I felt very invigorated by its energy.

I was beginning to impress myself with all these mental acrobatics when a new pain of mammoth proportions captured my attention and showed me who the real boss was. We had been taught a new meditation technique that required us to sit completely still for two hours without a break. About 1½ hours into the meditation, it struck me. I had just consumed two cups of coffee and a big bran muffin.

I now was not only experiencing excruciating pain in my buttocks that was intensifying with each passing moment, I felt like my bowels and bladder were going to spontaneously combust. Although that thought initially troubled me, after several more minutes of agony, I began to believe that spontaneous combustion might be a blessing.

After a few more minutes of intensifying agony, the moment of truth arrived. I decided to make a break for it.......I was going to the bathroom.

I planned each micro-movement of my journey with delicate precision. I felt like a mobster planning a bank robbery. However, the harder I tried to be inconspicuous, the more conspicuous I was. As I began making my way to the exit, the faint sounds of my warm-up pants legs rubbing together – which I had never noticed before – now sounded like thunderous roars. I felt like every eye in the meditation hall was watching me, and that if they failed to reach enlightenment, it would be my fault. Instead of getting any closer to my enlightenment, I felt like the spiritual police were going to whisk me away to spiritual Hell. The seventy-five feet between my seat and the exit seemed like light years.

By the time I got through the door, I could barely hold it in any longer. After sitting on the toilet, I had my *Nirvana* moment. When people said that Vipassana meditation can bring about Nirvana, I had no idea it would be like this.

That feeling of Nirvana, no matter how sweet it was, was very short lived. When I got back on my cushion, my old friend returned – this time more intense than before.

Instead of resisting it, I worked on loving it. I figured there was no better way to learn unconditional love than to learn to love something I intensely resisted. It is simple to love Mother Theresa or a happy day in the park. It requires unconditional love to love intense pain. I thought perhaps this unconditional love toward all that I'd been resisting was the necessary ingredient to finding Empowered Peace in The Zone.

The more I resisted in an effort to separate from the pain, the worse it got. Conversely, the more I accepted and merged with the pain, the less intense it became.

For the next several hours, I played with strengthening my equanimity with the pain. I got better at observing it from a place of no craving for comfort, no aversion, and no story. In this state of mind, time seemed to stand still, and there was an even deeper connection with everybody and everything. In retrospect, it felt as though I was in The Zone. At the time, if I had any such thoughts about what I was experiencing, it would have taken me right out of it.

The fewer thoughts I had, the less intense the pain became and the more euphoric I felt. The more I merged with the pain, the more intense the surge of energy I felt pulsing through my body.

This pain seemed symbolic of all the painful situations, evil people, and health challenges that had appeared as Frankenstein Monsters in my life. The more I merged with the pain, the more Bliss I experienced. No longer did anything feel separate from me. I felt the full implications of living in a non-local, **_non-dualistic_** world, the opposite of my conditioned **_dualistic_** way of seeing the world through the filters of thought. From within this non-dualistic perspective, there are no opposites, and everything felt interconnected. There is no such thing as pain and no pain, no "me" that is separate from anything else. Without the filters of thought, everything seemed to merge together into intense Bliss. As I left the meditation hall that day, the world took on a different character. I felt a deep connection with everything in existence.

Physicists agree that we live in a non-local Universe in which everything is interconnected. But this feeling of connection I experienced went far beyond what those theoretical words can express. I felt its implication in every cell of my body.

This experience brought about a dramatic shift. I felt as though I was watching a movie where suddenly everything changed from black and white to full 3-D Technicolor.

Although merging with the pain had brought about this shift, I still believed the pain might have even greater lessons that may not be learned by merely laughing at my thoughts.

No Thoughts, No Pain

As I moved deeper into this state, I found something miraculous. When I had no thoughts at all, I had no pain. At that point, I began to see the pain as a personal biofeedback machine, and my greatest teacher. It let me know whether or not I was thinking. As soon as a thought emerged, the pain returned. This realization helped keep me honest. Until this point, I believed that during most of the time I was meditating, I had relatively few thoughts. Now I realized I was just deceiving myself.

As the days progressed, I found this place of no thought was not only pain-free, but blissful beyond my wildest imagination. Somehow this excruciating pain had led me to what felt like a significant spiritual space I hadn't intended or expected to reach.

As the hours of sitting rolled on, I continued to discover different qualities of no-thought as part of my inner exploration journey. There was "active no thought," and a "passive no thought." "Active no-thought" seemed to be a more superficial level of no-thought, in which I was actively resisting thoughts. Then there was a "passive no-thought," a much more relaxed state of bliss that came from just letting go.

The more intense the pain, the more it forced me to go deeper into that place of no thought – into The Zone. It was as though I was doing Aikido, in which the attacker's momentum could be used to my advantage. I used the intensity of the physical pain to get deeper into The Zone.

From the place of no thought, some spontaneous thoughts seemed to emerge out of nowhere. They seemed very different from my usual thoughts – almost as though they were "God's thoughts." The main distinguishing factor between these thoughts and my usual thoughts was that these were generally loving, quiet insights that I would not ordinarily have.

Every time I had an agenda, such as to reach a state of ultimate Bliss, the pain would return with even more intensity, like a master punishing a rebellious disciple. I quickly realized that whenever I exerted my will, more pain resulted. So instead of exerting my will, I learned to surrender. When I did this, I had no discomfort at all.

Over time, as I went deeper into that place of no thought, it almost felt as if I had no mind and no body. All that existed was a feeling of Wholeness, within which an inner laughter started to bubble up. I began to laugh at the old way I had looked at myself as separate from the world. It seemed funny that I would have limited myself to being the space defined by the area where my skin ends. In this awareness, there were no longer any thoughts in place to delineate where I ended, and everyone and everything else began. Everything felt perfectly united as one whole being.

During some meditations, I found it extremely frightening to have no thoughts. When I had no thoughts, it felt as though there was no mind, no body and nothing to call "me." I felt as though I was dead. This feeling of death became overwhelming, to the point that tears fell down my cheeks. But when I surrendered to this feeling of death, the state of intense Bliss once again emerged.

It seemed as if that fear of death was deeply hidden under all my other fears, including the fears that had often caused me to run. Now, instead of running, I was sitting and realizing that, like the pain, this fear was hiding even more Bliss.

I began to laugh at the inconvenient realization that the pain I had spent my life studying and trying to eradicate in my medical practice could not only be eradicated, but could possibly be transformed into ultimate Bliss, by letting go of thoughts. I laughed about how this discovery could make some of my Medical training in pain management worthless once the cause of the pain is successfully treated. Freedom from thoughts seemed to lead to freedom from pain. I wondered if the technique would work for others.

The next day, I did a special meditation in which I focused my attention on the hollow space under the nostrils. As I did, I was drawn to focus infinitely more deeply. I found myself looking for the tiniest "Particle" in the absolute center of that hollow space under my nose.

It took quite a while to find that space, but after several more hours of meditating, I found it! When I fully experienced "The Particle," it felt like an atom bomb explosion of Peace, Love and what can only be called Absolute Bliss. In actuality, no words can describe that feeling, as it went well beyond the intensity of Bliss I had ever imagined possible.

Whenever I focused on the feeling of Bliss, it diminished. As long as I focused my attention on "The Particle," the Bliss continued to escalate to new levels. The potency of Bliss became so intense that it was difficult for the body to contain. It was so overwhelming, I thought if I let it go on any longer, I would begin making strange noises and possibly have a seizure. At that point, I defocused my attention away from "The Particle" to turn down the intensity of this Bliss.

As I meditated on other areas of the body, I found that they were different flavors of Bliss. The area at the bottom left part under the nostrils was hugely Blissful. The navel felt more like vast amounts of pure joy and love. I never imagined that contemplating one's navel could be so amazingly Blissful. It was so Blissful, I wouldn't consider trading that feeling for a million dollars!

It seemed that whatever area I meditated on was full of these atom bombs of Bliss, Love, and Joy at their core. I began to wonder: it seemed as though at the core - the essence of everything - lay not just atoms with protons, neutrons, and electrons, but also atom bombs of Bliss, Love, and Peace.

How ironic that in my previous efforts to resist pain, I experienced much worse pain and had unknowingly resisted experiencing this intense Bliss. My resistance to pain made it impossible to entirely stop and experience this absolute Bliss that was deeply hidden beneath my thoughts.

This revelation reminded me of the movie "My Fair Lady." It almost enticed me to break the silence of the meditation hall singing: "The strain in pain lies mainly in the brain!"

I later learned an accepted concept among some Nobel Prize Laureates is that we live in a non-dualistic world in which everything is interconnected. They say that we live in a world in which whatever we perceive is a mirror reflection of what is in front of it. From this perspective, it seemed funny that I was trying to resist my pain when, at some level, I was creating it. Although it appeared amusing that I would create such intense pain, it turned out to be the best gift and teacher I could have ever received.

I realized that, embedded within the dualistic way we perceive our non-dualistic world that is full of challenging people and situations and other Frankenstein Monsters is an **_Inconvenient Joke._** It was highly inconvenient to take responsibility for creating my pain, especially as a pain physician whose practice was focused on helping patients eliminate pain.

But, inconvenient or not, within our non-dualistic reality in which we are all interconnected, who else could I blame? I was essentially trying to blame my reflection and forgetting to laugh at how funny this would look to "God."

It seemed that within just about every thought was the implied belief that there is a world "out there" that is separate from me. This belief in separation prevented me from experiencing the Bliss that came from merging with everything, including my pain.

But once I dared to take responsibility for my reflection and had the courage to laugh at the contorted way I was conditioned to look at a non-dualistic world with dualistic thinking, the whole game I played on myself seemed very funny. It resulted in the miraculous transmutation of my intense pain to intense Bliss. This laughter seemed like The Ho-Ho Holiest Medicine there is. I wondered if experiencing pain and everyone and everything as separate from us, is the root cause of all the pain and suffering in the world. I wondered if laughing at this illusion of separation is The Ho-Ho Holiest Medicine.

God—The Misunderstood Comedian

I had been looking for God much of my life and thought that I had found Her during this meditation. I called this God, "The God of Laughter."

I thanked this God for helping me laugh at my contorted view of reality that resulted in this miraculous transmutation of intense pain into intense Bliss. This seemed like an Earth-shattering epiphany with tremendous implications. But this epiphany eventually resulted in even more questions.

Could it be true that "God, who sits in Heaven, laughs" (as it says in Psalm 2:4)?

Could H.G. Wells be right, "The crisis of today is the joke of tomorrow?"

Could God be a comedian who scattered "painful" people and events throughout our world waiting for us to find the hidden Joke?

Can laughing at pain, in whatever form it may take, enable me to begin to see pain from The God of Laughter's perspective?

Once I understand The God of Laughter's sense of humor, would I see God as a "Misunderstood Comedian"?

Would it be possible to transform the painful situations into Blissful ones by seeing the world through the eyes of this God of Laughter - as I did with my pain?

Once I laugh at my contorted way of seeing the world will I laugh along with The God of Laughter?

If I can heal my pain through laughter, and if our outer world is a reflection of our inner world, can laughter help heal our world?

I was grateful to the God of Laugher for gifting me with the perfect type of pain for this experience.

Note: Please know that some forms of pain may require other approaches that should be discussed with your medical doctor.

After the meditation retreat, I continued to marvel at how agonizing pains could transform to Bliss beyond description, with absolutely no medications and no change in the bodily condition.

I recognized that, whether I was trying to escape a corrupt government, pain, or any other Frankenstein Monster, there was no place to run, because the suffering was always originating in my inescapable mind.

It seemed funny that I had spent over thirty years reading, researching and traveling to distant lands in search of a guru, spiritual master or holy teacher, not realizing that the holiest teacher of all would be where I would never consider looking.

But if someone told me thirty years ago that my holiest teacher would be my holy butt and that I would find ultimate bliss in "The Particle" right under my nose, I would have told them to click their heels together three times, repeat "There's no place like home" several times, and to go back to Kansas.

While looking back and laughing at my past suffering, I began to appreciate the irony. I had spent much of my life running away from physical and emotional pain. It wasn't until I stopped running and struggling that the pain subsided into a state of Laughter and Bliss, well beyond what I had been searching for all those years. The Bliss was there all along, hiding in the most resisted experience, and in places I would never think of looking – my butt pain, and in "The Particle" right under my nose.

Perhaps the way to find this Bliss is to stop struggling......and start laughing.

My continued struggle to resist life reminded me of a Chinese Proverb:

A farmer and his son had a beloved horse who helped the family earn a living. One day, the horse ran away, and the villagers exclaimed, "Your horse ran away, what terrible luck!" The farmer laughed and replied, "Maybe, maybe not. We'll see."

A few days later, the horse returned home, leading a few wild horses back to the farm as well. The villagers shouted out, "Your horse has returned, and brought several horses home with him. What great luck!" The farmer laughed and replied, "Maybe, maybe not. We'll see."

Later that week, as the farmer's son was trying to ride one of the wild horses, the horse threw him to the ground, breaking his leg. The villagers cried, "Your son broke his leg, what terrible luck!" The farmer laughed and replied, "Maybe, maybe not. We'll see."

A few weeks later, soldiers marched through town, recruiting all the able-bodied boys for the army. They didn't take the farmer's son, who was still recovering from his injury. The villagers shouted, "Your boy is spared, what tremendous luck!" To which the farmer laughed and replied, "Maybe, maybe not. We'll see."

I spent most of my life on an emotional rollercoaster judging everyone and everything as good or bad, painful or pleasant, friend or enemy, running away from everything I judged as "bad," in my constant struggle to resist life. Now, after experiencing such intense Bliss after laughing at my excruciating pain I had so fiercely resisted, I wondered what other intense Bliss is possible if instead of resisting life, I laughed along with it.

In my continued quest to achieve the most dramatic, longest-lasting results by correcting the root causes of the pain, **I wondered if the deepest root cause of the pain and suffering in the world is our inability to laugh at *God's Jokes.***

"Be Realistic: Plan For a miracle."

— Osho

Chapter Four
The Paradigm Shift

I wondered, if I can tune into my idea of God's sense of humor and have a peak experience in the midst of excruciating pain during that meditation retreat, why can't I turn challenges into Bliss in my daily life? The shift from experiencing a torturing pain in my butt to a Blissful experience stayed with me as the source and a perfect example of this seemingly miraculous paradigm shift.

Understanding Miracles

I began to apply my new perspective to the idea of miracles. A fire-walk had a dramatic impact on my belief system several years previously. Seeing an enormous fire when I arrived, my first instinct was to turn around and run as fast as I could.

Before the fire-walk, we discussed how limiting beliefs influence our abilities. The leaders told the story of two physicians who did the fire-walk and had no blisters until five days later, when they got together for lunch to discuss the walk and the fact that the coals were over 1,000 degrees Fahrenheit. They agreed that it should have been impossible to come away from that heat without blisters on their feet, and within several hours of having that discussion, they both developed blisters.

During a pre-walk ceremony, we identified all our limiting beliefs about walking on fire, followed by a drumming ceremony to release those beliefs. The guides recommended waiting for our unique "window of time" – the time when we would Know we could do the walk.

I stood around the fire for what seemed like hours, waiting for my "window of time." I waited so long, that I was concerned the fire might go out and that my "window of time" would go out the window.

Then, the moment finally arrived when I Knew. It was as if an inner voice told me "now is the time." This realization was accompanied by a great sense of confidence and inner peace, knowing I could successfully do the walk. I did it with total focus and concentration. After completing the walk, I felt a massive rush of energy. I felt all fired up.

The day after doing my initial fire-walk I saw a patient who was on Morphine and had surgical instrumentation in his back after a lumbar fusion. I had never been able to help patients with these two complicating factors.

As I was about to tell him how sorry I was about not being able to help him, I felt a spark of inspiration. If I could walk on fire and not get burned because I had let go of my beliefs about fire, perhaps I could also change my limiting beliefs about Morphine and instrumentation and help this patient with the same miraculous conviction.

I treated this gentleman and am happy to report that he left my office pain-free and with a massive smile on his face.

I have done many fire-walks since then, and only had blisters on my feet once. To satisfy my skeptical mind about why these burning coals might not have caused any burns, I decided to walk on the coals while a bit closer to my usual state of mind, and without quite waiting for that perfect "window of time." Shortly after completing that walk, lo and behold, I developed blisters on my feet.

Miracles Greater Than These

The next several years were a turning point in my career. I developed a greater awareness of the impact of *my* thoughts, beliefs, and state of presence on *my patient's* outcomes. The walls that separated my consciousness from their health conditions became more fluid and flexible.

I discovered that whenever politics or distressing news stories were discussed during the treatment, any needles I used were much more painful, and the results not as good. As my equanimity and ability to practice medicine from The Zone increased, my results dramatically improved. **It almost seemed as though my ability to practice medicine from The Zone was more important than the actual treatment itself.**

I've used these experiences to form part of the basis for my medical practice. Over the years, I have seen many miracles with patients who failed to get better after going to countless other medical specialists and pain clinics, with various treatments including surgeries. Some of those patients had been in pain for more than thirty years, only to get their life back after several of my treatments from The Zone.

I began to think about the miracles *Jesus* had performed and how he said, "Very truly I tell you, whoever believes in me will do the works I have been doing, and they will do even greater things than these."

I had resisted the teachings of Jesus for many years. I was brought up Jewish and would have my mouth washed out with soap if I even mentioned His name. I eventually overcame this resistance because His profound and inspirational messages seemed to deeply resonate with me. His teachings allowed me to accept the possibility that ordinary people like me can perform miracles.

I began to wonder about the implications of these teachings. Could it be possible for ordinary men and women to perform greater miracles than Jesus? Could patients learn to heal themselves?

But when I began talking with other people about what Jesus said, they all had the same dumbfounded look on their faces, as if to say, "You're on planet Earth now. Get real!!!"

Since I didn't have enough facts on the tip of my tongue at the time, I probably had an equally dumbfounded look on my face, and quickly changed the conversation to the weather or the fantastic plays in last Sunday's Super Bowl game.

I became extremely curious about the science of miracles and how we could use miracles to change our lives and our world.

I was determined to understand God's Healing Humor and help others see the world from an empowered perspective. I wanted to address each person at the deepest part of their soul - the innermost part which innately knows the same truths Jesus described. I wanted my new treatment approach to be grounded and truthful, with facts anyone could easily understand and verify. I also wanted the information to be justified and substantiated by solid research. I spent many months investigating literature that yielded some astounding findings.

"If anybody says he can think about quantum physics without getting giddy, that only shows he has not understood the first thing about it."
— Niels Bohr

Chapter Five
The Science and Religion of Miracles

When I first set out to gather factual data as a basis for miracles, I was not very optimistic. I had read that miracles happen because the world we experience is an illusion of our own creation. But if that is indeed true, how could I prove it? Underneath that question, I had an underlying fear that if I could prove that everything is an illusion – such proof would also be an illusion; so why even bother?

I decided to ignore that troubling detail for a while because everything seemed confusing enough as it was. The possibility that nothing existed, and that there was nothing to be confused about, ironically, seemed even more confusing.

What surprised me was that finding the truth was easy. The tricky part was trying to get people to believe the truth when even I found it difficult to believe. I realized that I was so fixed in my beliefs that no matter how many facts I found, I preferred believing information that had been repeatedly disproven. I began to empathize with the Greek astronomers who lived over 2,000 years ago in their efforts to inform others that the world is round. But their job seemed simple in comparison to the job ahead of me. **I was finding that the world is neither flat nor round, but that it does not exist.**

It amazed me that confirmations of my new view didn't come from something written in the local psychic tabloids. These facts came from some of the greatest researchers who have ever lived, including Nobel Prize Winning Laureates, top quantum physicists, and Albert Einstein.

They also came from some of the core teachings of the most popular religions and spiritual texts.

Now I will share with you some of the scientific-based information for "left brain" dominant readers who want scientific proof for these seemingly radical conclusions about the nature of reality. This section of the book may challenge some right brain dominant readers. For this reason, I issue this light-hearted warning:

If your eyes glaze over, pupils dilate, or you turn a ghostly white; do not panic. As a medical doctor, my advice to you is to put the book down, lie down with your legs elevated, and take some deep breaths. When you feel normal again, you may want to skip to the next chapter, and revisit this one in the future, perhaps reading only one paragraph at a time. If any troubling symptoms persist, call your doctor.

The Joke of "Reality" According to Nobel Laureates and Scholars

Niels Bohr, winner of the 1922 Nobel Prize in physics said, "If anybody says he can think about quantum physics without getting giddy, that only shows he has not understood the first thing about it." When I first read that quote, I suspected Niels may have been taking some kind of Magic Mushrooms. Back when I studied physics as a pre-medical student, I experienced many emotions. Giddiness, however, wasn't one of them. But after digging deeper into quantum physics, I wondered if our consensus experience of reality is the most hilarious Joke of all.If some of the wisest people who have lived are correct, the only natural response to this reality is laughter.

The more I explored quantum physics in the context of how I lived my life, the giddier I became. The fact that Bohr was also giddy about quantum physics allowed me to feel justified in my giddiness and encouraged me to dig deeper into the Joke.

Albert Einstein said, "**Reality is merely an illusion, albeit a very persistent one.**" Einstein also said: "**Time and space are modes by which we** think and not conditions in which we live" and "Our separation from each other is an optical illusion of consciousness."

His words suggest that we live in an illusory non-local, **non-dualistic reality in which we are all interconnected.** We are spending our lives mesmerized by illusions and riding a roller-coaster of emotions that raise some people's blood pressure, or cause them heart attacks and strokes by responding to illusory stresses in an illusory reality that we call normal life and usual behavior. It's like a roller-coaster ride at Disneyland that made me quite Goofy.

A very crucial study was performed by French physicist Alain Aspect. He found that under certain circumstances, two sub-atomic particles that split and travel at the speed of light in opposite directions are always "in communication" with each other, regardless of how far apart they are. These subatomic particles can *instantaneously* communicate with each other, even if they were to theoretically move 10 billion miles apart. Somehow, each particle always seems to know what the other is doing. This study was repeatedly verified in other labs, including physicist John Bell's, and is what Einstein described as, "spooky actions at a distance." These studies serve as the basis of quantum entanglement and undermine what we believed about the nature of reality.

University of London physicist David Bohm believes that Aspect's findings of the two particles that communicated instantly, regardless of distance, is not because they are sending some sort of mysterious signal back and forth, but because their separateness is an illusion. If objective reality existed, it would be virtually impossible for the instantaneous communication to take place across such distances[1].

David Bohm said this implies that objective reality does not exist. Despite its apparent solidity, **the universe is essentially a gigantic and detailed hologram**[2]. This means that at some deeper level of reality, these particles are not individual entities, but are extensions of the same fundamental "something" in which **everything is interconnected** in a sort of "soup of consciousness."

The fact is, we live in a non-local reality described by many physicists. **The idea of non-local connections is not new-age fluff but is accepted in**

the scientific community. The hottest topic in modern physics is exploring non-locality. It was originally described by the saying "as within so without," but modern physics has finally caught up. The physicists are now taking over what was previously called metaphysics and parapsychology. Their work is now being published in premier mainstream journals. The validity of non-locality makes all the difference in the world. It is the reason that two sub-atomic particles that are 10 billion miles apart can influence each other. The reason is that in reality, they are not separate. **It is also how we may be able to transform everything from corrupt politicians to weather changes, and perhaps help heal our entire world.** Since everything is interconnected, when one interconnected particle changes, every else changes, sometimes in imperceptible ways.

Erwin Schrodinger, a quantum theorist who won the 1933 Nobel Peace Prize, said: "There is only one thing, and that which seems to be plurality is merely a series of different aspects of this one thing produced by a deception (the Indian Maya); the same illusion produced in **a gallery of mirrors**[3]."

This profound statement has been swept under the carpet, even though it came from Schrodinger, a Nobel Prize-winning Austrian physicist whose development of several fundamental principles in the field of quantum theory formed the basis of wave mechanics and formulated the wave equation. Schrodinger's assertion about the nature of reality has been virtually ignored because it doesn't fit with our concepts of reality. He was the author of many works in various fields of physics and was highly respected.

In fact, by ignoring the fact that we live in an illusory gallery of mirrors, we are ignoring our escape route from The Illusion. This ignor-ance is causing our suffering, as you will soon see.

It would be extremely challenging to accept the possibility that this world that seems so real may be one big illusion, if not for the other Nobel Prize Laureates who agree.

Niels Bohr was a Danish physicist who received the Nobel Prize in Physics and made foundational contributions to understanding atomic structure and quantum theory. He is quoted as saying, **"Everything we call real is made of things that cannot be regarded as real."**

It is tempting to read this last sentence and just keep going on a mission to finish reading this book by a certain deadline because it is inconvenient to consider its implications.

The irony of the implications is that, since everything we call real is not real, "nothing" is the only thing that is real.

I came to understand that, by regarding what is unreal as real, I was living my life acting like other people in this universal funny farm who also believe *their* illusions are real, and forgetting how funny this is. If "Martians" were to visit and see how berserk we look, they would quickly return to Mars and come back to Earth only when they were in the mood for more entertainment.

I thought that maybe the road toward sanity is to use my thoughts as a constant source of entertainment, but then had a concern. What if I were to laugh at each thought and those "normal miserable people" put me in a "funny farm" with other happy people who are labeled as "crazy," and they medicate me until I am as miserable as them? If this seems a bit confusing and is giving you a headache, you can thank God that your headache and this whole chapter are all unreal!

If this scientific side trip is a bit overwhelming or confusing, please feel free to skip to the next chapter, which should be easier for everyone to digest. But if you're still with me here, let's take a closer look at the nature of what we call "reality" and see if Powerful Laughter at the Cosmic Joke may be a logical response.

The Science of Oneness

Erwin Schrodinger said, "<u>**Subject and object are only one**</u>[4]." Schrodinger and Bohm both asserted that the separation between subject and object is an illusion, and that matter itself is a unified field without barriers.

David Bohm believes we greatly misunderstand the illusion of separation. He said that the whole Universe is in some way... **like a hologram,**

where each region of space-time contains information about every other point in space-time[5].

None of this made much sense to me until I did what Bohm recommended as a way of understanding this elusive holographic concept more clearly. I looked at the corner of a fish tank. As I stared at each corner of the tank, I noticed how each of the images was slightly offset and different. As I continued to watch the single fish that now looked like two fish, I became aware that when one turned, the other also turned; when one faced backward, the other also faced backward. If I was unaware of the situation, I might even conclude that the two fish must be instantaneously communicating with one another, when in reality I was only observing one fish.

It appeared as though there were two fish in the fish tank, separated by several inches, and moving in synchronous ways - just as there appears to be two particles in space separated by billions of miles. Ultimately, there is only one fish, there is only one particle, and indeed there is only one Consciousness that appears to be divided into everything we see and know.

The two particles in those Quantum Physics studies instantly communicated with each other because they are essentially the same particle, just as the single fish in the tank appeared as two. Along the same lines, different people may somehow be fundamentally the same essence, even though we appear to be separate.

Since there is ultimately only one fish, one particle, and one consciousness, once we dissolve our belief in separation, what was perceived as separate will eventually appear as one. This is where ancient spirituality and modern science also come together as one.

Werner Heisenberg's "uncertainty principle" and quantum theory both imply there truly is no objective reality "out there," independent of its relationship with the observer.

These geniuses were proposing there is no objective reality. Instead, there is an infinite number of possible "realities" - until our minds focus on one of them, bringing it out from what Bohm called the "implicate order" of oneness, and into apparent outer experiences of multiplicity.

This idea is further demonstrated in Schrodinger's famous cat experiment.

In this experiment, a cat is theoretically placed inside a closed chamber, in which there is a 50% probability of a radioactive substance being emitted. If the radioactive substance is emitted, it causes a flask of hydrocyanic acid to be released, and the cat is asphyxiated and dies.

Before the chamber is opened, the cat is "in superposition" – it is both alive and dead at the same time, with a probability of 50% for each state.

The point of this perhaps unnecessarily gruesome theoretical experiment is that the act of observing the cat as alive or dead is what puts the cat definitively into one of those states. Reality takes shape only at the time we observe it. In the absence of an observer, the cat may be both alive and dead at the same time.

This suggests that we have cause and effect completely reversed. It is our observation that "causes" the cat to be either alive or dead. In other words, our observation is the cause of the effect - of whether the cat is alive or dead. **This also means that we are the cause of our reality through our observation. This idea can help heal our world.**

This conclusion is further supported by Jim Al-Khalili, a nuclear physicist who said: "If you want to see fear in a quantum physicist's eyes, just mention the words, "the measurement problem."

The measurement problem states that an atom only appears in a particular place if you measure it. This means that an atom is spread out to infinity until a conscious observer decides to look at it. In this context, the act of observation can be said to have created the entire universe[6].

Since it created this universe, the observer can also theoretically modify it. This is known as the "observer effect," which says that **"the act of observing will influence what is being observed."** When this personal responsibility comes together with Powerful Laughter, miraculous healings can take place.

Believing our conditioned version of reality to be the only valid version leaves too many unanswered questions. "Reality" has been proven over and over to be dependent on an observer. How can anything that is real be dependent on an observer, unless it is the observation itself that brings "reality" into existence? And if we were to believe "reality" is real, it would be difficult to explain "The Quantum Measurement Problem," which shows how what is observed is dependent on the observer.

Quantum experiments have confirmed that there is no solid reality independent of the observer. What exists when we're not looking is a wavy cloud of infinite possibilities. It is only when we focus our attention on part of these waves of possibilities that infinite "reality" collapses into the "particle" of that possibility and becomes our personal experience. In this way, the act of observation creates the entire universe!

This explains why we're in such a mess. Instead of influencing our world in an empowering way, we think negative thoughts that are reflected back to us as a dangerous world, and we forget to laugh at what we and God's comedic routines are doing. Instead, we become mesmerized by our reflections, the "_**Illusory World**_" we call reality, and we suffer.

The great news is that since forgetting to laugh at The _Illusory World_ created our suffering, laughing at it may help free us from suffering, open the horizons of our perspective, and help us to heal ourselves and our world.

Once we stop and take the time to understand how we are behaving in light of the grand perspective of quantum physics and ancient spiritual philosophies, laughter may be the best and perhaps the only proper response to this incredible and humorous play.

Laughter – The Natural Response to a Reality That's Not Real

Albert Einstein said, "Time and space are modes by which we think, and not conditions in which we live." Powerful Laughter, which takes us out of thought, is a way we can transition from the time and space modes in which we've been conditioned to think - to a reality of freer conditions, in which we could, and ultimately do, live.

Despite all we know about the nature of reality being an illusion based on the findings of so many of the greatest scientific and philosophical minds, this concept may still be a bit difficult to swallow, as it was for me as I researched these studies.

The problem I had with all this information was that it just seemed like mind candy to a mind already bombarded with other conflicting information. I concluded that the only way for me to validate this theoretical view was by confirming it for myself.

I validated it for myself by recalling and applying quantum physics to my Vipassana experience, in which I experienced no pain when I had no thoughts.

When I had any thoughts, I experienced pain. Since the thinking mind does the observation, when I had no thoughts, there was virtually no observer present to experience any sensation.

I essentially had my own experience of Heisenberg's "uncertainty principle," which implies that there truly is no objective pain "out there," independent of its relationship with the observer.

Without any thoughts, I had no pain. I, therefore, must have thought my pain into existence. And just as I thought my pain into existence, it is possible that we think ourselves into existence. This may be why Descartes said, "I think therefore I am."

Some of the things we think into existence may need to be tamed, like my pain. One way to do this is through equanimity and calming our thoughts. Another way is by laughing at our thoughts, essentially laughing at the Cosmic Joke that can be hilarious and terribly inconvenient at the same time.

Since reality is an illusion and we can tame our mental lions with Deep Inner Peace and Powerful Laughter, it would follow that equanimity and laughter would restrain our ability to harness our anger. One concern I had while considering a complete loss of anger was that it could hamper our ability to harness the power of anger that so often fuels our efforts to make necessary changes.

However, using the power of anger to make changes can also lead to a potentially slippery slope with adverse side-effects. While we may be trying to harness anger, that anger often harnesses us and takes us out of The

Zone, out of the space of True Power. To me, the only solution seemed to be to wake up from the Illusory World.

Although this reasoning seemed like a sound scientific and experiential basis on which to support the importance of **_waking up_** from the Illusory World, I was curious to learn what religions, philosophies, and ancient scriptures had to say on the topic.

Reality According to Religion, Philosophy and Sacred Scriptures

Immanuel Kant is a German philosopher considered by many to be the greatest modern philosopher and a major influencer of contemporary thought, especially in the realm of metaphysics, ethics, and political philosophy. Like Einstein, he said that "**Space and time are not attributes of the physical world.** They are modes of human perception. They are powerful lenses of our own invention, and they often serve to limit our experience....That is, they act as lenses that block us from perceiving true reality[7]."

Plato's allegory of the cave is one of the best-known, most insightful attempts to explain the nature of reality.

The tale is about prisoners living in a cave, chained so tightly they cannot even turn their heads. All they know of reality are the shadows in front of them projected onto the cave wall by puppeteers behind them.

Since they cannot move their heads and these images are all they've ever known, they naturally presume the images to be real. Because this is the only reality they've ever known, they believe that it is normal to suffer and have adapted to this version of reality.

Eventually, one of the prisoners manages to break free from his chains. As he approaches the entrance to the cave, he sees sunlight. At first, he is blinded by the light and unable to comprehend this experience of a world outside the cave.

As he turns back toward the cave and peeks inside, he realizes that the figures on the wall that had been his total impression of reality were merely shadows.

In an effort to enlighten the other prisoners, the freed prisoner goes back to share this newly discovered knowledge of "reality." But the prisoners are so set in their habitual way of thinking they don't want to hear the true nature of reality by someone who is free. Not only do they think he is insane, but because he threatens their version of reality so much, they want to kill him.

The cave represents the state of most humans. The tale of a dramatic exit from the cave is analogous to entering a greater understanding of reality beyond our previous limitations and illusions.

The idea of the world being an illusion is not a new one. "*Maya*," "*Lila*" and "*Samsara*" are the names given to this illusion in ancient times.

According to **Hindu** philosophy, the world is nothing but "*Maya*," which is Sanskrit for "illusion."

Eastern philosophies are based on the awareness of a unity and mutual interrelation of all things, people, and events. This ultimate indivisible reality which manifests itself in all things, and of which all things are parts, is called *Brahman* in **Hinduism**. In **Buddhism,** it is called *Dharma-kaya*. In **Taoism**, it's called *Tao*, "The Way."

In the story of **_Adam and Eve_**, the apple can be interpreted as a metaphor for *Maya*. By swallowing the apple, mankind metaphorically swallowed the lie that the world we see is real. This is considered by some to be the "original **_sin_.**"

In **Christianity,** Jesus said, "I and the Father are One" and "Very truly I tell you, whoever believes in me will do the works I have been doing, and they will do even greater things than these." Since Jesus miraculously healed the sick, we should be able to do "even greater things than these."

Jewish mysticism says much the same thing in the teachings of the Kabbalah. The Kabbalah defines the nature of humans, the nature and purpose of existence and the nature of **reality**.

Its central book, the Zohar, is an ancient sacred scripture. It serves as a guidebook to the lost divine nature of our souls. It is a collection of virtually all information pertaining to the universe; information that science is only beginning to verify today. The Zohar says that our physical world is an illusion, a temporary residence, and **not true reality**. It is essentially a dream.

Vedic literature agrees that the plurality we perceive is only an appearance - not reality. It says, "Even though apparently awake, one is still asleep if one sees multiplicity."

Taoists emphasize the paradoxical and interdependent nature of dreaming and so-called "reality." Chuang Tzu, a famous Taoist, said, "Someday comes the Great Awakening when we realize that this life is no more than a dream ... The great Confucius and you are both a dream. And I, who say all this is a dream, I too am a dream."

Ramana Maharshi was an Indian sage who radiated peace and contentment. He was known to many as the silent sage whose peaceful presence and powerful gaze changed the lives of those who came into his presence. He said, "The difference between a dream while sleeping and the dream we call wakefulness is only of duration, one being short and the other being long."

For **Buddhists**, spiritual life is about Awakening from the dream of unreality. The word Buddha itself derives from bodhi, which means "Awakened." Buddhist spiritual practices are designed to Awaken us from the daydream of illusion and confusion, where we are like sleepwalkers, semi-consciously muddling our way through life.

The Buddhist sacred text the *Flower Ornament Sutra* says, "The mind is like the master painter" that paints our reality.

The Illusory World

In summary, objective reality does not exist. The act of observing will influence what is being observed. There is no space. Separation is an illusion. Everything is One and <u>what we call our world is merely a holographic, Illusory World consisting of a *Hall of Mirrors* appearing as a dream from which we have not yet Awakened. It is a dream in which perhaps the mind can be seen as the master painter of our "reality."</u>

Our sleeping and waking dreams are merely different forms of dreams in which the "waking dream" is a dream from which we have not yet **_Awakened,_** and therefore have yet to recognize it as a dream. All the miraculous experiences and all the pain or pleasure we experience during a dream can seem just as real as those we experience when we are awake.

From our sleeping dreams, we realize that our minds can experience things that seem completely real. It is only after we Awaken that we realize everything in the dream was merely a creation of our own minds which we mistook for reality.

In some ways, the world we believe as real is like a holographic image. When a holographic image is projected, we can actually walk around it and see it in three dimensions from different angles. It looks very solid. One of the most fascinating properties of a holographic image is that when we, for example, cut a holographic image of a rose in half and magnify the images, we find that exactly the same full image of the rose is seen in each of the halves. If we then cut those halves into halves again, we find the same thing. This process can continue infinitely, and we will still see the same image in its entirety in each piece, though from smaller three-dimensional angles. Each part of a hologram contains all the information within the whole, yet it is all an illusory projection of laser lights shining through photographic plates.

The holographic nature of the Universe is verifiable in our life. We see examples of reflected patterns wherever we look, from electrons spinning around an atom's nucleus to the planets spinning around our Sun. In many healing modalities, the ear, foot, and eye are used as holograms for the rest of the body. The deeper we investigate this, the spookier it gets!

It's like in a dream where we travel thousands of miles. All that distance we seemed to have travelled, and all the dramas that seemed so real in our sleeping dream actually took place in the space between our ears. Similarly, the distance and separations we experience in the "waking dream" world are also occurring in the space between our ears.

This analogy helped me understand how all separation is ultimately an illusion. It validated my Vipassana experience and brought about a profound shift in the way I looked at the seemingly separate world around me. After having these insights, I thought about the words of Jesus, "And you will know the truth, and that truth will set you free." I wondered whether these findings were the truths that will set us free from the Illusory World.

As Jesus said, "As above, so below, as within, so without." What is outside of us is a hologram for what is inside us. Our body and its diseases are a hologram of what is going on in our mind.

That is why it is said that God created man in His own image; man is a hologram of God.

The most important teaching of many spiritual paths is to "Know Yourself." When we know ourselves, we know God.

God can create miracles. Once we accept the fact that reality is an illusion and we *Know God* by *Knowing Ourselves*, we will truly understand what Jesus meant when He said that we will do even greater things than Him. We will then be capable of miracles, of self-healing and things more magnificent than we'd ever imagined.

We doubt these possibilities as a result of habit and our cultural conditioning. We ignore even the idea of being able to do greater things than Him. For some reason, even Christians tend to trust their cultural conditioning more than these teachings of Jesus. Instead, we believe a disempowering philosophy borne of ill-informed cultural conditioning, rather than the empowering teachings of Great Ones such as Jesus.

Note: If you skipped ahead and your color has returned to normal, and you have a pulse, you can resume from here.

No Time, No Space – Just Laughter

In conclusion, everything I read from the Nobel Laureates geniuses to religion, philosophy and ancient sacred scriptures seemed to be saying what Einstein summed up so succinctly, "Time and space are modes by which we think, and not conditions in which we live." None of these quotations were intrinsically funny, but as I kept these quotations in mind and observed how we live our lives, they could seem hilarious.

Since, as Einstein said, time and space are not conditions in which we live, everything is happening here and now, within the One Mind of which we are all a part. There is no separation between people, animals, places or things because for such separation to exist, space would need to exist to create that separation.

Some of us spend our whole lives angry, regretful and guilty about the past - and worried, anxious and fearful of the future. It is a never-ending battle to resist something we don't want or crave something perceived to be outside of us. Our "success," which is always right around the next corner, would enable us to someday live happily ever after, as was "proven" over and over in fairy tales. We forget to laugh at how funny this all is because most of what we do is based on a belief in time and space, which may be the biggest unlaughed at Joke in history.

As will be apparent by the end of this book, the more I investigated this Inconvenient Joke, the funnier it eventually became. As you also may laugh about after finishing this book, this world is essentially a holographic **_Hall of Mirrors_** in which every single mirror reflects some unique aspect of us. Like a dog barking at his multiple reflections barking back in a house of mirrors, we believe all these evil Monsters outside of us (in the mirrors) are out to get us. The whole concept of a separate entity that is outside of us would require space - which, according to Einstein and spiritual sages, does not exist!

Laughing at The Inconvenient Joke is so inconvenient because it forces us to admit that we are the ones causing those terrifying images to look so frightening. Instead of being like Jesus and doing miracles greater than Him, we scare the beJesus out of ourselves, until finally, if we are fortunate, we **_wake up laughing_** at ourselves for taking this whole charade so seriously.

This new kind of Laughter led me to these questions:

1. If the mind is like the "master painter" who paints our reality, is it possible to use this paintbrush to experience miracles?
2. Could laughing at the Inconvenient Joke help empower us to help heal us and our world?
3. If this is possible, how can I make it all happen?

"Very truly I tell you, whoever believes in Me will do the works I have been doing, and they will do even greater things than these."
— Jesus Christ

Chapter Six
The Miracle of Laughter

A Course in Miracles says that a miracle is a correction in perception. It removes the blocks of fear and guilt, allowing glimpses of timeless joy. Let's explore whether this correction in perception may be achieved through laughter and whether it can open the doorway to experiencing miracles in our lives.

One night I was tossing and turning in bed while trying to devise a fun way to change perception without needing to meditate long hours or reading piles of spiritual books. I kept hearing those same words of Jesus in my mind, "I tell you the truth, anyone who has faith in Me will do what I have been doing. He will do even greater works than these." I also kept hearing other seemingly outrageous words of Jesus, "And you will know the truth, and that truth will set you free."

These words seemed to imply that I can experience miracles greater than Jesus if I have faith in Him and know The Truth. But then I began to wonder, "What is the Truth?"

Lao Tzu said, "The truth that can be spoken is not the real truth." Although that definition seemed rather limiting, it all began to make sense.

My Vipassana experience caused me to realize that any thought, or as Lao Tzu would say - any truth that can be spoken - corrupted my experience of Bliss. Could I experience that Bliss as a byproduct of embracing the "Real Truth" - the Truth beyond thought, and if so, how?

I began to wonder:

1. If the "Real Truth" was what I experienced during my Vipassana meditation when I had no thoughts, could this be a way of transforming intense pain into Bliss?

2. Are there miracles and Bliss all around us waiting to be experienced once we let go of conditioned thoughts?

3. Could we experience miracles and Bliss as a natural part of life, once we laugh away these conditioned thoughts?

4. Since laughter leads to the place beyond thoughts, can Powerful Laughter help us find miracles and Bliss without needing to meditate?

Inspiration for the Cover of This Book

I held onto those questions for the next several months, until one night during a sweat lodge ceremony, when I had another life-changing experience.

My intent during the ceremony was to access that Blissful state I had tasted during my daily life and to experience miracles. The result seemed to be just the opposite, as I almost died during this process.

To get the most out of the ceremony, I sat near the heating element of the sweat lodge and didn't take breaks. As a result, I felt the most extreme intensity of heat. The intensity of this discomfort was similar in many ways to the extremes of pain I'd experienced during Vipassana.

The intense heat brought me to an altered state of consciousness. In this state, I saw a never-ending grid of what looked like zeros and ones, which seemed to be the basic building blocks of my ordinary reality. This grid had an overwhelmingly terrifying and Hellish feel to it. I felt lost in it, without a world to hold on to.

Although I could see a way out, I had no idea how to get there. I saw how with each thought, I had created each pixel of that grid. I also saw how my thoughts were creating my Hell, and how the totality of that grid represented my reality.

Then, out of nowhere, one of the others in the lodge began laughing. This laughter slowly spread to others until there were waves of infectious laughter that continued spreading. This laughter felt so transformational that I was overwhelmingly confident that laughter is a necessary ingredient to make shifts in consciousness that can profoundly change our world.

Within the juxtaposition of this laughter and my overwhelmingly terrifying experience of this **_Illusion of Hell_**, I felt as though there was a big Joke that I didn't quite understand.

From that experience of laughter within the Illusion of Hell, I saw a major shift taking place as we surrendered to a state beyond thought – to a state of laughter.

This experience made me wonder if there could be a Grand Comedian, who seems extremely cruel but may be tremendously Loving once we understand and Laugh at His Jokes. I also wondered if Powerfully Laughing along with "The God of Laughter" can open "The Door" - to take us from the world created by our conditioned thoughts - to God's world of Heaven on Earth.

It was this experience that inspired the front cover of this book.

Toward the end of this experience, I felt like I was given a profound informational download of answers to every imaginable question. This allowed me to experience reality from the perspective of being interconnected with all of reality. It helped me experience who I really am in a way that cannot be described in words. It was a perspective in which "Do unto others as you would have them do unto you" was completely redundant and quite funny because the "other" was indeed me. It was a perspective from which all wars, corruption, lies, and beliefs in scarcity disappeared into perfection. This reality seemed more in alignment with what "God" intended than my ordinary reality. In juxtaposition with my unquestioned, unconscious belief that we are all separate, this download seemed hilarious, and I couldn't stop laughing. It seemed hysterical that despite being perfectly interconnected parts of the same humongous organism, we play a game on ourselves of competition, anger, and fear of annihilation, forgetting to laugh at how funny this is.

Because I was so caught up in this laughter and I didn't take any water and fresh air breaks, toward the end of this experience, I eventually became unconsciousness. Because the sweat lodge was pitch black, no one realized my state until I had been unconscious for quite a while.

I felt as though I had not breathed in quite a while. I now had the opportunity to choose whether or not I wanted to take the next breath. I chose to breathe, without giving it any thought.

When the others in the sweat lodge finally realized what had happened, they tried to revive me with fresh air and gallons of water. Although I had a vague awareness of my surroundings, I was unable to talk or move for several hours. After several more hours, I was able to move but completely unable to understand words or move without assistance. Several hours later, I was able to put together some thoughts. That was a mixed blessing because it included the haunting thought about how I could be living as an invalid, entirely dependent on others.

Despite being semi-conscious, I realized I needed to use my few remaining functioning brain cells. I realized that the only way I was going to return to my normal life was to completely focus on what it looks, sounds and feels like to be completely healthy as my only possible reality. I used the maximum intensity of pure focus I could gather.

I did this for the remainder of the night and into the morning. I woke up with intense thirst and intense pain in my leg but was able to function almost normally. Having no idea what that pain was coming from, I looked down at my leg and saw an extensive burn completely down to the bone.

My leg had apparently been resting on the heating element in the sweat lodge for quite a while, yet I was entirely oblivious to this intense burn because I had been nearly dead.

Laughing at the Illusion of Hell

Over the next several months, I felt that something major had shifted. I had an improvement in my intuition with my patients, beyond even what they were aware of. My fear of death disappeared, and I tended to laugh a bit more when confronted with challenging people and situations. I felt calmer and more loving, even toward those I would have negatively judged in the past. I also experienced a shift in priorities away from traditional goals and more toward my spiritual evolution.

My near death and Vipassana experiences had given me a glimpse of what life is like outside the Illusion of Hell; a Hell that until now I believed was a normal part of being human. Even though I thought I had everything I needed and was relatively happy, I had no idea of how miserable I was compared with how I felt during those experiences.

I had acclimated to this Hell, like a frog being scalded to death in a pot of progressively hotter and hotter water. I had no idea how much I had been suffering in the scalding waters of this Illusory World of Hell until I jumped out of the pot. Now, I was determined to jump back in and help others in their escape. These experiences and determination served as a basis and motivation for this book.

Laughing Like Our Lives Depend On It

Despite how Blissful it felt to take this peek outside my Illusion of Hell, I knew my work had just begun. I felt as though I had been born again with a new purpose in life – to help myself and others break out of our Illusions of Hell.

But the more intent I became on making this great escape, the more questions arose:

1. How do we escape something that seems so invisible and so much a part of being human?
2. If it is true that what we resist persists and gets stronger, how can we escape or resist anything when the act of trying to escape causes that thing to be more difficult?
3. If I were able to escape, how would I be able to relate to other people who were still mesmerized by their Illusory Worlds?

One of the major realizations I had from my near-death and Vipassana experiences is that my thoughts are creating my illusion of what I now saw as Hell. I found that even my best thoughts within The Illusion could not compare to the magnificence of that state beyond thought.

I concluded that the way to escape is by achieving a steady experience of that Blissful state beyond thought. This would involve letting go of conditioned thoughts by laughing at them.

While pondering the question of how to escape anything when the act of trying to escape causes such escape to be more difficult, I thought about a story. Two soldiers were about to kill each other with their automatic rifles when suddenly, they heard a helicopter overhead. Soon afterward, they see M & M's of all different colors and fillings raining down from the sky. One soldier says to the other, "I'm starving, and those M & M's look delicious. Let's throw away our rifles and eat those M & M's." The other soldier says "Sure, I don't know why we are fighting this war anyway." They eat the M & M's and live happily ever after.

I thought, maybe laughter is like the M & M's. Maybe laughter can allow us to let go of old thoughts and transform war into peace. Perhaps it can help us transcend the Illusory World of Hell created by conditioned thoughts, and live "happily ever laughter."

Over the next several years, I dabbled with Lao Tzu's quote, **"As soon as you have made a thought, laugh at it."** Those eleven words seemed more profound to me than anything else.

That Lao Tzu quote also provided a possible answer to my old question: How do I escape the Illusory World, something that seems so real and so much a part of being human? I realized the way to experience that Bliss is by noticing, laughing at, and unraveling the factor that was blocking that experience – which is thought. I had no thoughts when I experienced that profound Bliss, so conditioned thoughts seemed like the main obstacle to this Bliss. I discovered that Laughter unravels thought by a process we will discuss in detail later.

Lao Tzu's quote also might work in tandem with Einstein's: "We cannot solve our problems with the same thinking we used when we created them." What better way of solving problems than with an activity that is not only a different way of thinking, but takes us to a state beyond thought? And to make Laughter even more attractive, it's an activity that doesn't require hundreds of hours of meditation or even a single dollar – and it's fun to do.

Lao Tzu's words could provide the tools necessary to bring that state of Deep Inner Peace into daily life because it takes us to a place beyond thought. Since cravings and aversions are the causes of our suffering and are created by thought, what better way of letting go of suffering than by laughing those thoughts into oblivion? This is very exciting! Laughing at thoughts could lead to freedom from them and be a yellow brick road to lead the way out of the Illusory World!

Because laughter is of very high vibration, when we laugh at our most negative thoughts, we instantly and radically raise our vibration and attract people and situations that match that vibration.

Laughter, The Detergent to Clean Away Suffering

Laughing at our thoughts is like putting them into a washing machine and getting rid of their emotional charge. As we continue laughing at The Inconvenient Joke, we may notice progressively fewer, less frequent and cleaner laundry, until the only things remaining are God's gifts.

Laughing at our thoughts is a way to eradicate suffering in the world. This is because there is a huge difference between pain and suffering. Pain, whether physical or emotional, is a pure sensation. Suffering results from the thoughts about pain. Those thoughts that cause suffering can be cleaned away by laughter.

This laughter is not a way of "making light" of a bad situation. It is a way of breaking free from the emotional bondage brought about by our unlaughed-at thoughts.

Disclaimer: Just like there is no one medicine for everyone, laughter is not for everyone. Some people may prefer being angry and depressed about life's challenges. I am not here to take that away from them, but to show them another option.

From my Vipassana and near-death experiences, and in my daily life, I found it helpful to challenge each fixed belief, preferably by using laughter to bypass the mind.

That is how our fixed beliefs.......actually become fixed!

The magic of Laughter goes well beyond the experience of laughing. It is a soulful experience that brings us to the space beyond thought. Without the filters of thought, we are better able to feel our connection with everything in existence.

We can think of emotions as the audience for our thoughts. When we have positive thoughts, we have positive emotions. Those positive emotions cause us to emit positive vibrations that are reflected back to us as a positive world. Laughter creates positive vibrations by creating a positive train of thought. This Laughter train has destinations beyond what we may have thought could be available.

Many people spend a great deal of effort engaging in mental exercises, trying to raise the vibration of their thoughts by one emotional level at a time. Many consider it easier to go in steps from revenge to anger, or from pessimism to boredom than to go directly from anger to joy. But what if we can jump directly from anger to laughter? Depression to laughter? Suffering to laughter? Throughout this book, you will find tips, examples, and discussions about how and why this process is possible and enjoyable and can happen at the speed of thought.

Laughter is like the clutch in a car. If we are in low gear, laughter disengages that gear and allows us to cruise along in a higher gear. The more we laugh, the higher the gear. Imagine what would happen if many people around the world made laughter an integral part of their lives for generations to come.

But, before we get too excited about the power of laughter, I need to make some points clear:

- **Laughing at our thoughts as soon as we think them may be extremely difficult.** If it were easy, this would be a one-line book. Nevertheless, by the time you have finished reading this book, you will have the tools necessary to remove the blockages to laughter and lead a happier, healthier and longer life. Even then, this laughter will take ongoing practice which can take many years to become a permanent change.

- **Laughing at thoughts does not condone any action.** We are laughing at our <u>thoughts</u> about what was done, not about <u>what</u> was done. This allows us to take action from a space beyond thoughts, cravings, aversions, behaviors, habits, and programs. We act from a space more connected with our Higher Self, in which we have access to more creative ideas about how to change our conditions. Some may call this "acting from The Zone," or from the "God Space."

- **Everything I say in this book is also a thought, and therefore fuel for laughter.** Don't believe anything I say before laughing at it. Whatever thoughts remain after your laughter, you may want to hold onto for a while as long as you keep the laughter going. If in doubt what to think or do........just laugh!

With all this said and after writing this book, admittedly, I also find it challenging to laugh at many thoughts. But I find that I am progressively improving and feeling better the more I practice.

Just like the day to day practice of many spiritual traditions can be challenging, the practice of laughing can also be very challenging. The advantage of laughing over other spiritual practices is that it is more fun and it doesn't create additional cravings or aversions, which may create additional blockages to living in The Zone.

Since many happy people have found that "enjoying the journey is the goal of the journey," we might as well choose a journey that is fun.

Laughing at Everything

Lao Tzu said, "The Tao that can be spoken is not the eternal Tao." Nothing that can be written or spoken is true. Many beliefs our ancestors held as true were subsequently proven false. Many beliefs they held as false were proven true.

Our ancestors were absolutely convinced that the world was flat, and might have thrown you to the wolves for suggesting otherwise. In fact, there are still people called "flat-earthers" who insist that the globe we've seen in so many photos from space is somehow flat, and the center of everything. Our predecessors would have thought it impossible that someone could talk into a rectangular device and immediately speak with someone thousands of miles away. That idea might have gotten some visionary women in Salem declared as witches.

Of course, if nothing written is true, Lao Tzu's quote must also be false. Perhaps everything written and spoken is meant to be fuel for our laughter, after laughing at that thought as well.

Even if all I have written in this book is entirely false, and even if my theory is no more valid than the Tooth Fairy, I invite you to take a moment to consider how you feel when you believe it is true versus when you don't. Consider how your emotional well-being is affected by the difference. Which do you choose right now, knowing you can change your mind whenever you like?

Even though we know the people, places and things we see in a movie are coming from a projection booth and may be based on a story that is completely fabricated, we suspend our disbelief to enjoy the movie. What if we can also go on a similar adventure into the depths of laughter? What if we can temporarily suspend our disbelief, take Lao Tzu's advice, and laugh at our thoughts, laugh at everything in this book, laugh at our life, and experience the different perspective this Laughter brings?

What if the only benefit of this laughter practice is to enable us to experience more peace, more joy, and better health, from a place one step closer to The Zone?

How we can get into The Zone is a topic discussed throughout this book. For now, suffice it to say that perhaps we get there by going the opposite way from the way we left it. According to *A Course in Miracles*, "Into eternity, where all is one, there crept a tiny, mad idea, at which the

Son of God remembered not to laugh. In his forgetting did the thought become a serious idea, and possible of both accomplishment [the separation happened] and real effects."

This means that we were in the Heavenly experience of our Oneness with God when we wondered what it would be like to no longer experience Heaven. We forgot to laugh at that idea, got lost in the illusions, and wound up where we are now.

Many believe the original sin is our belief in our separation from God and Our Wholeness. I believe the real original **sin** is our forgetting to laugh about how this separation can ever be possible. Our return to this Heavenly experience of Wholeness happens by remembering to laugh at how ridiculous the notion of anything other than Heaven can be. It also happens by recognizing that we are always connected with the Wholeness of God, in a Heavenly state that often seems to be obscured by conditioned thoughts. That Heavenly state is experienced again when our conditioned thoughts are washed away with laughter.

The Sweet 16 Reasons to Laugh at Our Conditioned Thoughts

1. To Wake Up to a world beyond our limiting thoughts and beliefs, and beyond our wildest imagination.
2. In order to live in a Heaven on Earth, it is helpful to laugh away our limiting beliefs that are preventing this from happening.
3. Laughter has the power to make big problems seem smaller and easier to handle.
4. Laughter allows us to heal our thoughts and beliefs, which is key to healing our reality.
5. Trying to second guess 'God' with the tunnel vision of our pee-wee brain is funny.
6. Laughing at our thoughts turbo charges our evolution. It helps us achieve a state of Deep Inner Peace wherever we go, which could take decades of meditation or many decades of therapy to achieve.

7. Laughter comes naturally once we realize how funny it is that we diligently try to change our reflections without even considering the possibility of changing what is being reflected.

8. The popular book of spiritual transformation called A Course in Miracles refers to laughter 43 times. It essentially says that forgetting to laugh causes us to believe the Illusory World is real. We may infer from this that perhaps laughter is the way out.

9. Why suffer when we can laugh at our thoughts that create the suffering?

10. Laughter feels good.

11. Laughing at our challenges can be a fun and creative process where the real challenge is – how can we reinterpret the situation in an empowered and funny way (which we will discuss in Chapter 20)?

12. If we could be anxious or depressed by all the traumas and dramas in our world, or see our "traumas and dramas" as the greatest comedy skit on Earth by laughing at our thoughts about them, which would you choose?

13. Laughter is a miracle – a correction of perception that corrects thoughts and takes us to the realm beyond thoughts and into The Zone – to our place of Power.

14. Laughter allows us to Awaken from The Illusion and function in The Zone.

15. If laughter really is the best medicine, why not take several daily doses?

16. After contemplating all these reasons, why not laugh at the reason that we don't need any reasons to laugh?

Another reason to laugh at our thoughts is because they contradict the teachings of the wisest and most spiritual people who ever lived. Despite how much those people say that we are a Divine, interconnected soup of consciousness, we behave as though we are being victimized by some of the soup's ingredients. Because we become attached to the way the soup should taste, we whine. We forget to laugh at secretly wanting flavorful and exciting soup, and that perhaps - the whine belongs in the soup.

Despite Jesus saying, "Whoever believes in me will do the works I have been doing, and they will do even greater things than these," we behave like the grown elephant who still believes it is incapable of breaking free of a flimsy rope tied to a post after trying unsuccessfully as a baby elephant. We are essentially roped in by our limiting thoughts and beliefs. We forget to laugh at how funny these thoughts would seem if we were to tell them to Jesus - who said we will do things greater than Him.

Reasons Not to Laugh at One's Thoughts

- If I laugh, people might think I am crazy.
- It's a habit not to laugh.
- Most thoughts are not funny according to the mind (which has a vested interest in keeping thoughts and the resulting Illusory World alive).
- If I laughed, the whole Illusory World would be in grave danger. Since my entire world is filtered through thoughts, if I laughed them away - I would be totally disoriented and would have no way of making sense of my experiences.

As we look at those lists, doesn't the list of reasons to laugh seem much more appealing?

Another factor to consider is that when we laugh, we shift our biochemistry, and therefore our health. It may be difficult to eradicate a tumor or create a normally functioning heart, but we can always change our thoughts about them. Since our thoughts are the co-creators of our reality, as we shift our thoughts we shift our reality.

It may be tempting to not laugh at positive thoughts, but as I found in my Vipassana experience, even the most Blissful thoughts prevented me from experiencing the ultimate Bliss I experienced when I let go of even those thoughts.

By laughing at our thoughts, we are releasing the obstacle that is interfering with our ability to witness miracles. Laughter at all thoughts may be our causative miracle that unblocks God's miracles.

Accessing "The Zone" to Experience Miracles

To understand how it may be possible to experience miracles, let's first determine what a miracle is.

The word miracle comes from the Latin *miraculum,* which is derived from *mirari,* to wonder. A miracle, then, is an event that provokes wonder. A miracle appears unexplainable. It is in some way contrary to our expectations and may appear to be caused by the power of God.

A Course in Miracles says that a miracle is a correction in perception. Through that change of thought, miracles can happen. A miracle "does not create nor change anything at all." Since the world reflects our perceptions, and since perceptions are a product of thought, nothing needs changing other than our perception and thoughts.

What more fun way of changing our perception and helping us synchronize with God's world than learning how to laugh at Her Jokes? This change in perception can help create miracles because, according to quantum physics, we attract what resonates with our vibration. As we correct our perception to align with God by laughing at Her Jokes, we enter The Zone, where we attract what appear as miracles.

The Zone

The Zone is a Superman-like state. It allows elite athletes and others to feel as if they are invincible.

I've heard many stories of people who have accessed this Superman-like state. Tony Cavallo was repairing a 1964 Chevrolet Impala that was propped up with jacks. While he was working under the car, it fell on him. His mother, Angela Cavallo, miraculously lifted the car high enough and long enough for two neighbors to replace the jacks and pull Tony from beneath the car.

Lydia Angiyou saved a child by fighting a polar bear until a local hunter shot it.

There are many similar stories of people who access The Zone to perform what we consider miracles.

I accessed The Zone during those long hours of Vipassana meditation when I broke free from my thoughts into entirely new realms of awareness. The Zone is available to anyone; it is the place where passion, excitement, and determination meet equanimity. The easiest approach to accessing The Zone is by laughing at our thoughts.

The Zone is a state of intense single-mindedness and complete immersion in the present moment, where there is such complete absorption in an activity that the activity itself is intrinsically rewarding and other needs become negligible. It is the ultimate state of harnessing emotions in the performance of an activity. The Zone is experienced as pure focused motivation. This state is then positively energized and aligned with the activity in a timeless complete state of flow. There is no trying, only effortless movement, without thinking. It is always accompanied by a spontaneous feeling of absolute Bliss. There is the complete loss of a separate self, and the experience of time is altered. It is a state from which miraculous self-healing can happen. This is the state from which much of this book was written.

To be in The Zone requires the complete loss of a separate sense of self; it is a state where we let go of our conditioned beliefs of separation and embrace the Truth that we live in a non-local reality in which we are all interconnected.

Let's take a moment to consider the implications of this interconnectivity while practicing medicine in The Zone. Think about how it may be possible for health practitioners to be more successful in helping to facilitate the miraculous healing of their patients, even at a great distance, by practicing medicine from The Zone.

Anyone can enter The Zone and help heal themselves and the world. All it takes is the ability to laugh at our thoughts and to laugh at the Inconvenient Joke.

"The crisis of today is the joke of tomorrow."
— H. G. Wells

Chapter Seven
The Inconvenient Joke

I invite you to join me on a journey. Let's put on a special pair of imaginary _x-ray glasses_ that allows us to see beyond our conditioned way of experiencing reality. These glasses would enable us to see reality in alignment with the conclusions of history's greatest scientists and our world's greatest spiritual teachings. They would allow us to see the Cosmic Joke hidden within everything in our imaginary world. They will show us why This Joke is so inconvenient but necessary to laugh at. These glasses allow us to laugh at The Joke, and laughing at The Joke enables us to step outside the Illusion of Hell.

Einstein said, "We cannot solve our problems with the same level of thinking that created them." Since we create our reality with our collective thoughts, which help create our chaotic world, let's see if we can change our way of thinking, or use laughter to help let go of our thoughts, to help heal our world.

The reason for putting on these imaginary glasses is that our traditional way of seeing reality does not make any sense considering what we know from Nobel Laureates. Also, as you may have noticed, it doesn't seem to be working very well. Our traditional ways of seeing reality are responsible for most of the chaos and suffering in our world, because they are based on the illusion of separation. When we perceive "others" as separate from ourselves, we tend to judge them. We sometimes make them wrong and worthy of our attack. This can eventually lead to much of the chaos in the world.

Once we laugh at our thoughts about separation and embrace our unity, we will treat others as we would have them treat us. Once we do, much of the chaos in the world will disappear.

It seems a bit humorous when we realize how seriously we take this illusory reality. Even though we know that reality is "a gallery of mirrors," a non-local grand illusion, we insist on taking this illusion very seriously. We think it is normal to believe The Illusion is real, yet we put people away in padded cells for believing *their* illusions are real.

Our preference for illusions may be explained by the same taste for drama that inspires us to pay money to sit in a dark movie theater watching the illusions projected onto a screen. Because if you thought the quantum physics in chapter five was boring, just imagine how bored we would be living in a world described by physicists, in which there was nothing except empty space. That reality would make watching trees grow on slow motion videos seem exciting. If nothing else, this Grand Illusion is quite entertaining. And once we begin to access The Cosmic Joke, it will keep us laughing heartily, whether our current life illusion movie is a comedy or a tragedy.

This entertainment also allows us to explore the depths of **Who We Really Are** by observing the reflections we see. Once we put on these imaginary glasses, we see the world as a holographic Hall of Mirrors.

The more we laugh at our thoughts about our illusion of separation (instead of getting lost in the Holographic Hall of Mirrors that appear to confirm our belief in separation) we allow the hologram to be a graphic illustration of our Wholeness.

Laughter at our thoughts and the Inconvenient Joke is a profound way to unify humanity, by letting go of divisions created by the mind and mutually agreed-upon illusions. Laughter respects different religions and spiritual beliefs.

Separating from Our Belief in Separation

The cause behind anger and any war that causes people to suffer may be that we forget to laugh at our erroneous belief in the illusion of separation.

It is very easy to miss our essential unity because it is culturally accepted and widely reinforced that the illusion of separation is real.

We also have invested so much in this version of reality that it becomes inconvenient to let it go. Everything we have done since the day we were born makes up this investment. Because of this investment in The Illusion, it is inconvenient to put on those special glasses of unity.

Without these glasses, we continue to see the world through the filters of conditioned Belief Systems, the beliefs we have unconsciously acquired from those around us from the day we were born. This false worldview has been handed down for centuries. Sorting through each of our misconceptions would be extremely difficult. But the good news is that, once we see the Truth through these glasses, we can at least appreciate the humor.

One possible way of trying to make sense of this perception of separation is by reinterpreting the "Big Bang" in a different way. What if the tiny mad idea of the possibility of separation was responsible for the creation of the Big Bang?

The "Big Bang" may have occurred in two different ways – on a universal level and on an individual level. Before the Big Bang, everything was in a state of perfect Oneness. The Big Bang started the transformation of that Oneness into the potential illusion of separation. On a global level, the Big Bang occurred billions of years ago at the conception of the universe. On an individual level, the Big Bang is the cosmic magic that sparked our soul to take birth.

To say that the resulting illusion of separation is responsible for suffering may seem like a bit of an overstatement until we realize that this belief in separation is responsible for competition, jealousy, greed, and the underpinnings of most hostility and wars. The Big Bang is responsible for causing us to see Frankenstein Monsters in the form of certain people, situations or diseases which are out to get us. Instead of falling for the traumas, we can tear off those Frankenstein masks with the awareness of this non-local reality within which we are interconnected. We can see those Monsters as another part of us, showing us our blockages to wholeness.

But, rather than being thankful for our Frankenstein Monsters for showing us our blockages to wholeness that were responsible for the Big

Bang of the Illusory World, we often feel like giving them a Big Bang.....on the head! And judging from the Monsters' flat heads, perhaps someone beat us to it!

Instead of working on ourselves to integrate our fragmented selves, we are continually distracting ourselves with television, shopping, and even reading spiritual books about forgiveness and unconditional love. We seem to have an unconscious belief that the more we learn about spirituality and the more workshops we attend, the more spiritual we will appear to our friends, and the better we will look in God's eyes.

I gained a lot of knowledge about forgiveness and unconditional love. I had been an excellent student and could impress many people at dinner parties with all my knowledge, but I had not applied it in any serious way in my life.

Little did I know that the way to let go of divisions could seem so simple, yet can be so challenging: laughing at The Inconvenient Joke!

This laughter may seem very difficult in this challenging world full of Frankenstein Monsters, until we see those Monsters from the perspective of our interconnectedness and we laugh at our perception of separation.

Dr. Bloom's Allegory – A New Model of Reality

One way to authentically laugh at The Inconvenient Joke and begin to unravel our belief in separation is by considering the following allegory:

Imagine floating up to the Heavens. As you look down, you see yourself sitting in front of a Hall of Mirrors. You can see yourself going through your whole life chained in a virtual cave, with a Hall of Mirrors in front of you. You are chained in a way that keeps you from even turning your head. All you know of reality are the images in the mirrors directly in front of you.

Right behind you is a lens, and behind the lens is a very special Light: "_**The Light of God.**_"

Since you are chained so tightly and have been unable to turn your head, and since you have looked into the Hall of Mirrors for your entire lifetime, all you know of reality are the reflections in those mirrors.

At the beginning of your life, your lens was clear, and the reflections in the mirrors reflected back to you a Heavenly world full of Divine miracles. As the years progressed and you came out of alignment with this light, the lens became more and more distorted, causing the reflections in the mirror to become more and more distorted.

Initially, the reflections looked Blissful and had glowing smiles on their faces. But as the lens became increasingly distorted, the reflections seemed more and more sad and distorted, eventually becoming more ugly and frightening, until they began looking like Frankenstein Monsters.

In this cave of a limiting worldview full of fear, you spent your entire life trying to make those Monsters look happy, but they continued to look very frightening. At the same time, their reflections were so intoxicatingly fascinating that you were mesmerized and entirely entranced by them, absorbed in the drama of believing that those frightening creatures were out to get you.

Then, after reading the teachings of the wisest men who ever lived and using your x-ray glasses to observe yourself in front of your Hall of Mirrors, you make a fascinating discovery.

It suddenly becomes obvious to you that the reason the reflections are becoming distorted and looking more like Frankenstein Monsters is because the lens behind you – the lens that once transmitted the Light of God - is distorted. You realize that every time you have any aversions or cravings for things to be different or resist the flow of life in a way that causes any negative emotions, you have fallen out of alignment with the "Light of God." This results in more distortions in your lens.

The more mesmerized you become with those images, the more you forget the Heavenly experience of being perfectly aligned with the "Light of God" in a world full of miracles. You believed that if you tried hard enough, you could make the reflections look happy. You believed you could create a happiness that was better than the way you felt before you fell out of alignment with the Light of God.

Because you were so mesmerized by the world of reflections, and this world seemed to make so much sense to you, you continued to play the game, hoping that one day all the reflections would smile, and you could live happily ever, just like in the movies. Because this game was so fascinating, and you didn't know what would happen if you stopped playing along, you decided to continue. Because your family, friends, and community were all playing the same game, you were afraid to tell them about your discovery - afraid they would think you were crazy for questioning their own mad illusions.

You may have assumed that if the world were found to be just a Hall of Mirrors, that news would have surely made headlines in the Herald and there would have been regular bulletins from the BBC, CNN, and Fox News.

But you didn't realize that the people who are reporting the news are also your distorted reflections within the illusion of the holographic Hall of Mirrors. They are merely reflecting your fascination with playing the game.

In some ways, the Hall of Mirrors sounds a bit like Plato's Allegory of the cave that was written around the year 520AD, before the knowledge of quantum entanglement - the influence of an observation on what is being observed – was understood. But in Plato's allegory, the prisoners had absolutely no control over the shadows they saw on the cave wall.

In my allegory, however, the observer is completely empowered, because the reflections are a direct response to their thoughts. Unlike Plato's Allegory in which the prisoners are victims of their reality, my Allegory suggests that we "prisoners" are the creators of our reality.

According to my allegory, we are not *the* creators, but rather the *co*-creators of our reality. Our reality is co-created along with God/The Power of God/All That is/The Universal Energy/The Light of God/The non-local collective/non-dualistic mind - all represented in my allegory as the Light behind the lens.

We may never know the true nature of reality, but we can come to understand Erwin Schrodinger's assertion that "Subject and object are only one" and that what we experience as reality is like the illusion produced in a gallery of mirrors.

My Allegory is a way to incorporate Schrodinger's teachings into your daily life. As you will see, it has the potential to make the difference between living in Heaven or Hell. Nobel Prize laureate Jean-Paul Sartre (who refused to accept the award saying that "a writer should not allow himself to be turned into an institution") said "Hell is other people." We live in a collective Hell because we believe of the unquestioned belief in the illusion of "other people." This belief is so pervasive, so secretly powerful, and so much a part of how we interact with our world that to question it may seem irrational. Just about every sentence in the English language contains a pronoun. These *__pronouns__* strengthen the illusion of "other." Yet we continue living in a Hell created by all the implications of living in a world of "other people." Once we realize what we are doing, and use the tools described in this book to laugh our way out of this Hell, we can live in a Heaven on Earth.

My Allegory is one way to use the Frankenstein Monsters in our daily lives in order to help us break out of our collective Illusion of Hell.

Why go through life with disempowering beliefs that contradict quantum physics, especially after considering that these disempowering beliefs result in a disempowered reality? Why not embrace the empowering realization that we are the masters of our world and learn how to navigate within this truth through Powerful Laughter?

In my Allegory of the Mirrors, the "Light of God" represents the will and power of God, which can provide us with a Heavenly world full of miracles. When we stop distorting this light with our noisy thoughts, its beauty is reflected back to us in our mirrors. This pure light can enable us to experience Heaven on Earth – full and absolute Peace, Love, and Miracles. The more we live our life in The Zone, the more we align with this Light, and the more we align with this Light, the more we can live our life in The Zone.

We can come out of alignment with this Light of God any time we resist a person or situation or have a craving for things to be different from the Will of God. It is okay to have preferences for things to be different and take the necessary steps to make our aspirations happen. But any time we are not entirely present and in a Deep State of Peace with the way things are, any time we refuse to laugh at our thoughts and get pushed out of The Zone, we come out of alignment with the Light of God.

We come out of alignment with the Light of God and create distortions in our lens whenever:

- We tell or live a lie.
- Believe the Frankenstein Monsters in our Hall of Mirrors are out to get us.
- We are out of alignment with our authentic self – the part of us that Knows what is right and what would bring the most Love into the world.

The distortions in our lens represent all the times and all the ways our thoughts, emotions, and feelings have been out of alignment with the will and the Light of God. Ways to laugh away these distortions are discussed throughout this book.

The Easiest Way to End Wars, Terrorist and School Shootings

Our conditioned beliefs cause us to feel separate from the Light of God and separate from each other. They also cause it to appear as though our Frankenstein Monsters are out to get us. Because of this Inconvenient Joke we play on ourselves, we feel anger toward others. Some who have personality aberrations may even wish to destroy their imagined Monsters through wars, terrorism, or mass shootings.

If children were taught The Joke in grade school, the rule of "treating others as they would treat themselves" would be completely redundant and unnecessary. It would make the military and police useless. Imagine the possibility of a day where children who heard about a school shooting or nuclear war threat would know these events must be taking place in a science fiction movie. This potential future is a real possibility once we laugh at The Joke and see others as our reflections.

The same Hall of Mirrors that creates illusions can also allow us to see distortions in a way that enables us to heal them. Once healed, we are again aligned with the Light and Power of God. When we are most aligned with this Light of God, we are our true, authentic Self, capable of experiencing more miracles.

Forgetting a Minor Detail

The Joke is that we have forgotten a minor detail that changes everything, which is that we have cause and effect reversed. What we may perceive as a problem is essentially part of a bigger solution. The Frankenstein Monsters are helping to jar us awake. They are also providing us with valuable information about the nature of our distorted thoughts that need healing. We are playing this Joke on ourselves, but because this Joke is so enormous, so mesmerizing, so constantly reinforced by the media and everyone else who is not laughing, we forget it's a Joke.

Instead of working on changing ourselves, we insist on trying to change our reflections, forgetting that our reflections will never change unless we change first. We forget to laugh at how we continue using the same approach, expecting a different outcome each time, and blaming God for not changing our reflections. We continue to believe that if we try hard enough, one day our reflections will smile back at us, even though we are frowning. We forget to laugh at ourselves for this ongoing charade and forget that if we would laugh at our thoughts, our reflections will have no alternative other than to laugh back. But because we don't understand The Joke, we continue to suffer and set ourselves up for scary reflections.

It may seem inconvenient to laugh at this realization because doing so would shatter our whole perception of reality. But once we see through this entire charade and laugh at it, we regain control of our Hall of Mirrors. There is no need to fear that our reflections may get angry at us for putting them out of business, and all the devastation our lucidity may bring. Once we face these fears and laugh them away by remaining completely conscious of how these and other fears were created, we have escaped our Illusory World.

This "Joke" may seem like the product of a very sick sense of humor to someone who has cancer, chronic pain, and other health conditions, or someone behind on their mortgage payments or whose ex-husband is verbally and physically abusive. This "Joke" may make even the worst night club comedian's material seem hilarious.

I am certainly not going to invalidate any disgust you may have toward the suggestion to see even bad things through the lens of The Joke – that's why it is called an Inconvenient Joke. I'm just here to give you another way of looking at your life that may be empowering. This perspective can help you feel much happier and is based on scientific information and ancient philosophies. I am here to help you see the power of your thoughts, and help you recognize the Joke of your perceived limitations from an empowering perspective. All that is required of you is to have some curiosity about how this may be possible.

If you are curious, it is important to understand my allegory that I just described, as I'll be referring to it often.

It may take months or even years to be able to laugh in the face of challenges. I am confident, however, that by the end of reading this book you will have the necessary tools. From then on, it will take ongoing practice to laugh at The Joke and your thoughts wherever you go. It doesn't matter how long it takes. What matters most is that you enjoy the process. By enjoying the process, it won't seem as long, it will be more effective, and will be much more fun.

For now, let me just say that if you're not already laughing, it may be because you see yourself as the person mesmerized by your Hall of Mirrors.

Yet, every time we laugh at the Inconvenient Joke and at our thoughts and emotions, we are taking another step closer to the exit from the Hall of Mirrors. Our laughter is also helping us live in a state of Deep Inner Peace that is a necessary ingredient to living in The Zone.

The Inconvenient Joke may not sound funny, but if we take the time to step back and completely let go of our conditioned way of seeing the world from a perspective that is more aligned with the ideas presented earlier, we can begin to appreciate the humor. So please, just take a deep breath, sit back and relax. I am confident that if you follow the suggestions, by the end of this book you will see your challenges from a more peaceful perspective. You may even find it extremely convenient and empowering to laugh at The Joke.

Our perspective of challenges may change from an "awful" one, to one that is "awe-full" – one that is full of awe; one in which we are a-mazed by a maze of illusion.

Because we forget to laugh at The Inconvenient Joke, we tend to go about our daily lives as though nothing has changed, even after knowing about it. It is as if we are living with a pink elephant in the living room. We see the consequences of The Joke wherever we turn, yet fail to see the elephant that is responsible for it. It is not as if the elephant is trying to be incognito, wearing dark sunglasses and a camouflage negligée. We don't see it because everyone we know who is "sane" refuses to see the elephant. Ignoring this elephant is why it takes so much energy to be "normal."

Although our refusal to see the elephant is certainly taking its toll, the exact "change" necessary to pay the toll is laughter at the Inconvenient Joke.

Many of us refuse to laugh, insisting on taking the Joke way too seriously, just as we do with our nightmares.

There's a story about a woman who had a recurring nightmare where a Monster was chasing her. She would frantically run away from it, in a state of absolute terror. One night she was barely managing to stay ahead of the Monster when BAM! - she hit a wall and there was nowhere to go. The Monster caught up to her and the woman cried out, "Oh no, what am I going to do?!" The Monster looked at her and said, "I don't know lady, it's YOUR dream."

We are convinced by the "sane" people around us that it is normal to frantically run away from our Monsters, forgetting that these Monsters are merely reflections. The more we ignore them, the more out of alignment we become with the truth, the more distorted our lens becomes, the scarier our Monsters become, and the further and more frantically we need to run.

As we watch ourselves diligently trying to change our reflections, we find that in so doing, we have cause and effect completely reversed. We are utterly convinced that whatever happens in the mirror affects us. We are completely oblivious to the fact that our thoughts, beliefs, and emotions are the cause of our reflections.

We keep trying to change the reflections while ignoring their cause. For years, we have believed that we are victims of our world, when we are the co-creators of it. It's time to wake up to the realization that *we* are the cause of our reflections. We've had cause and effect completely reversed. We have to turn our usual ideas of cause and effect upside-down.

Such a minor detail, but such an enormous result. It's a good thing we can take a Joke!

The Greatest Magic Show on Earth

This Joke results in the greatest magic show that has ever existed. Just as by using misdirection, a magician causes you to focus your attention on the sexy women in bikinis while he creates the illusion of pulling a concealed rabbit out of an empty hat, misdirection is used to make us focus our attention on the Hall of Mirrors rather than ourselves. The dramas misdirect our attention away from where all action originates – divine light flowing through the universal lens and makes us ignore the elephant in our living room. This misdirection keeps The Illusion alive until we are ready to laugh at this Inconvenient Joke.

This elephant in our living room is composed of all the facts that we ignore, including facts about how reality is a non-local gallery of mirrors which is a grand illusion. Intelligent thinkers have tried to tell us about this illusion by saying:

- "There truly is no objective reality "out there," independent of its relationship with the observer."
- "Separation of each other is an optical illusion of consciousness" in which "subject and object are only one."
- "Reality is merely an illusion, albeit a very persistent one."

By ignoring these facts, we come out of alignment with the Light of God, and we suffer.

We are the greatest magicians of all time. **Instead of the ordinary magician who creates the illusion of pulling a rabbit out of their hat, we pull an entire illusionary universe out of the space between our ears.**

One way to break out of the Illusion of Hell and see reality for what it is, is through laughter and by using our Frankenstein Monsters as our teachers.

We have the choice of seeing our Frankenstein Monsters as evil people who must be resisted and destroyed or seeing them as the shadow parts of ourselves that need healing, parts of us that we have ignored and resisted. They are our greatest teachers - meant to help us regain our Wholeness. The Indian sage Sri Ramakrishna went so far as to claim, "The play is enlivened by the presence of troublemakers. They are necessary to lend zest to the play – there is no fun without them."

Frankenstein Monsters are like the excruciating buttocks pain I experienced during my ten-day meditation retreat. Instead of seeing the pain as my Frankenstein Monster and suffering, I saw it as my greatest teacher and experienced Bliss beyond words.

I believed my Frankenstein Monsters were out to get me until I began laughing at myself for not seeing how they were my greatest teachers.

Sometimes it takes a great deal of soul searching to see how our Frankenstein Monsters are our greatest teachers. **But if we search and laugh enough, we enter a massive epiphany in which everything gets turned upside-down, and an "ah-ha-moment" becomes the "ha-ha moment."**

Laughing Too Hard: Oops—The Disappearance of the Universe

If we take the time to continually dive into that ha-ha moment, we find some interesting ramifications, including what may appear to be an eradication of the world! For in that moment of complete laughter, with nothing remaining to be laughed at, the world as we know it will have served its purpose.

Although the disappearance of the Universe may sound like the perfect solution for getting rid of all the chaos and animosity, when we really think about it, this disappearance would be highly inconvenient for the evolution of our soul. Without a universe, we would not know Who We Really Are or how to experience the kind of profound peace that can never be taken away, regardless of our external circumstances and degree of global chaos.

To experience that Peace, we need the world and other people in our life to play different roles; the difference is that in Peace, we understand that everyone including ourselves is playing apparently separate roles within ultimate Oneness.

To learn how to find that profound peace, we subconsciously attract people that challenge us. One way to explain how this works involves a process that is helpful for people who have done life-between-life hypnotic regression – the belief that we make an agreement with everyone "else," each one signing a contract to play their required roles.

Everyone has agreed to take their role very seriously, and we all agreed to do our very best to try not to laugh because if anyone were to laugh, the whole charade would be over.

After we were born, a grand hypnotic spell was cast over us to cause us to forget why those people and challenging situations would be in our life. But after doing some deep soul searching or hypnosis, the laughter may strike. We may discover that the people and situations we have faced over our lifetime were the perfect ones to force us to use all our skills in order to experience a profound peace that can never be taken away from us, despite the most challenging conditions.

Once we have faced and laughed at all the Frankenstein Monsters that have been necessary to teach us all the lessons we need for the evolution of our collective soul, the Universe as we know it can disappear.

Laughing Away Old Memories

There is a story of two sages who were walking along a road. The road led them to the Ganges, a place where the river was chest deep, and there was no bridge. As they were about to wade through, a beautiful woman came up and said to the older sage, "Please carry me across to the other side."

The younger sage looked wide-eyed at the elder sage and said, "Don't do it! We are sages, what have we to do with women?"

The older sage said, "That's right, but this poor lady is pregnant."

"Pregnant or not, it is no business of ours. We must not so much as touch a woman!"

The older sage smiled, shrugged, and said, "Anyway, I will help her."

The younger sage was dismayed. "Well, if you want to fall into sin then don't let me stop you."

So, the sage carried her on his shoulders. They crossed the river, and when they were safely on the other shore, he put her down, and they went their separate ways.

For about two miles, the two sages walked in silence. The younger sage became increasingly agitated. He finally couldn't help himself and said, "It was awful that you carried that lady across the Ganges on your shoulders. Awful!"

The older sage responded, "I left her back at the riverbank. We have already walked two miles, yet *you* are still carrying her?"

Unhelpful memories are like the pregnant woman. We may carry them for quite a while in our minds instead of addressing the need they bring and laughing them away.

One reason it may seem so difficult to laugh old upsetting memories, thoughts, and emotions away may be due to karma. Karma is the principle of cause and effect where intent and actions of an individual (cause) influence the future of that individual (effect). Karma is based on the physics of our reality.

Perhaps *we* were an evil Frankenstein Monster to someone else when we were younger, or maybe in a past-life incarnation. In that scenario, the Frankenstein Monsters that are currently in our life are giving us the opportunity of working off this negative karma by laughing at the old hidden actions and memories that have resulted in this karma. We should be thankful for this opportunity; however most of the time we have a sense of resistance toward these Monsters. That resistance can further complicate the situation and create even scarier Monsters and negative karma until we finally become grounded in The Joke and can laugh at even the most terrifying Monsters imaginable.

If, instead of laughing away our memories responsible for our karma, we choose to resist our "enemy," we may run into even more obstacles, like a comedy of errors and Monsters showing up everywhere we turn. Since the world we experience is a reflection of us in the Hall of Mirrors, the more we resist any "enemy" that appears to be outside of us, the more out of alignment we become with the Light of God. The greater this misalignment, the more distortions are added to our lens, causing our Frankenstein Monsters to look even more frightening, and creating fear, anger, agitation, and despondency. This is the reason for the popular saying that "what we resist persists." The result of all this resistance is to make the Inconvenient Joke even more inconvenient.

One can think of the most "evil" people in the world as being the result of our collective karma as a society. It may be tempting to rejoice in the belief that the "evil" people will eventually be punished as a result of *their* karma. But since we are all One, when we wish punishment on others, we unintentionally create more distortions in our lens, and scarier Monsters take visible form.

Instead of wishing for karmic retributions, we can see the whole situation as a grand karmic dance. Most of our Frankenstein Monsters are looking for different dance partners to make the dance more exciting, and often find that the people who resist them the most are the most exciting dance partners. As soon as we notice these motivations within our partner, we can choose to pull the plug on the music, call off the dance, and with that, the dance would be over. We call off the dance through love and forgiveness, and by laughing at this whole game.

Calling Off the Dance

For many years, I believed that if I called off the dance by giving the Monsters in my life love and forgiveness, they would have a party and do the cha-cha all over me. But several years ago, in my private medical practice, I had a secretary who became a great teacher, when she triggered me to become fuming mad after she acted aggressively and confrontational. I was afraid of asking her for anything because I was terrified of her response.

One day I decided to forgive her for her behavior and appreciate her for her Cosmic role. I also chose to speak with her - allowing my words to come from a loving and compassionate heart.

Her responses ranged from being dumbfounded and astonished to relaxed, peaceful and more than happy to do whatever I asked.

Another time I called off the dance was when a wave of patients canceled their appointments at the last minute. Standing around for hours while waiting for my next patient to arrive infuriated me immensely especially after hours of preparation for their consultations.

Then one day when I had several cancelations, I decided to stop resisting and used that time productively and was amazed by the result. No sooner did one patient cancel than a new patient scheduled. It almost seemed as if they had somehow coordinated my schedule even better than it had been planned.

The more I've looked, the more this Joke seems to be the recurring theme. All my Frankenstein Monsters repeatedly infuriate me until I laugh at my thoughts about them and essentially call off the dance. Once I do, instead of Frankenstein Monsters, I see them as my laughter teachers.

It may still be a considerable challenge to laugh in the face of intractable diseases and at corrupt politicians. But remember, **we are not laughing at the situation, we are laughing at our thoughts about the situation.** While a situation may seem beyond horrendous because of our thoughts and judgments about it, after laughing at our thoughts enough, we may finally see the situation from the "God Space." From that God Space we may realize, as Albert Einstein said, "God doesn't play dice with the Universe."

Although we may not be able to see the purpose of challenging situations from our very narrow perspective of reality, the more we laugh, the more we may become aware of their grand purpose. Perhaps that purpose may be to work off karma from a past life, maybe to bring up lessons in forgiveness, unconditional Love, or genuine laughter that need to be learned, or even to allow people to die and join their loved ones in Heaven.

Having highly charged thoughts and resistances to someone is a by-product of the original sin of seeing others as separate. This sin gives rise to the illusion of separation from everyone and everything around us and causes the arising of fear and conflict. When we feel love, compassion, and gratitude for our Frankenstein Monsters, we will be one giant step closer to our freedom from suffering and liberation from the Illusory World.

It may seem difficult to feel love and compassion for our Frankenstein Monsters until we realize that corrupt politicians, tyrannical bosses and many of our Frankenstein Monsters derive most of their power from our fear and resistance. Whatever we resist not only persists but grows stronger. Therefore, any political resistance movement needs to see how their approach may be increasing the strength of their perceived opponent.

<u>Please hear me clearly. I am not saying we should allow our Frankenstein Monsters to continue with their victimization. I am saying that whatever we do, we make sure it comes from a powerful place of choice. We should do whatever it takes to resolve the situation, as long as this action is coming from a place of love and compassion, for the greater good of all concerned. When we do that, we move from resistance to acceptance and align with the power and miracles of God.</u>

Laughing at Corrupt Politicians

By withdrawing our intense fear and resistance against corrupt politicians, bosses, or others with power, we are taking away their power and allowing them to change, or for the situations to transform. Just as fear and resistance fuel our Frankenstein Monsters, love, compassion and laughter destroy them. Offering them love, compassion, and our hearty laughter is like throwing water on the Wicked Witch of the West.

Corrupt politicians and their leaders consist of only about one percent of those who run a world. Along with the seemingly never-ending supply of news stories eliciting fear and resistance, the way they maintain their power and Neilson ratings is by telling us shocking stories about "others," whether Muslims, Communists, Blacks, or Whites, to foster more division – a strategy that is designed to divide and conquer. We continue playing along with their destructive games until we wake up to the fact that within our non-local reality, division is impossible.

If we believe the stories that promote separation and division, we take a big step back from peacefulness and happiness into the illusion of suffering, separation, and disempowerment that is waiting to gobble us up like a shark-filled moat around a beautiful castle. Once we let go of our belief in separation by unconditionally loving all our most frightening Frankenstein Monsters, we reclaim our power as an integral, co-creative part of the whole. As you'll see in upcoming pages, I've been through this process several times, including with one politician who was so repulsive to me that I packed up and moved out of the country, only to eventually return to America to face my Frankenstein Monsters head-on after writing this book.

Our job is to remember that so-called corrupt politicians, health challenges, and all our other Frankenstein Monsters are illusions that are showing us the distortions in our lens. Our job is to give them love and compassion - and to laugh at The Joke.

Just as we do at night in dreams, we have concocted a great script of this world. It is full of trauma and drama, just like one of those old Alfred Hitchcock horror movies. Yet, because we enjoy the drama so much, we continue eating our popcorn and getting more and more sucked into the plot. The anxiety subsides when we wake up, finally realizing that it's just a dream.

Let's face it, despite all that has been said about the illusory nature of reality, this movie looks very real to most of us. Asking someone to love the most "evil" people in the world because someone said we are all connected may be all that's required for some people to understand. But that is not the way most people see it, despite anything they've read.

One way of understanding the nature of reality is by letting go of the desire to ever understand it. This is because any understanding must come through the filters of the mind, fueled and driven by thoughts and words. The problem is that the mind is incapable of understanding the nature of reality because it relies on the filters of thoughts and words.

When looking at a map, the United States looks as if it is separated from Europe by the Atlantic Ocean. If there were no water in the ocean, we would see that they are indeed connected.

Likewise, it looks as if people are separated from each other by thin air. We think the air between us creates that separation, but this notion is more a function of how we use language to filter our perceptions of reality. We believe that because the air is a separate entity and are a different entity, there must be separation.

Our words and thoughts create our beliefs in separation - which results in our grand illusion of separation. When we let go of those beliefs, we can see and experience that, within the interconnected soup of consciousness, no such separation exists.

It may seem difficult to deny that other people appear to be separate from us because what we see is filtered by the mind. But our eyes continuously lie to us. They are a product of our Belief System, which as you know, is a bunch of BS.

As discussed earlier, we can also see how our eyes lie to us when we look at a fish from the corner of a fish tank. Even though there appears to be two different fish moving at exactly the same time, in the same way, there is only one fish.

Similarly, the illusions of separation look a bit hokey and fishy. It can cause us to flounder and lose our soul.

Although we appear as separate bodies separated by containers of skin, we are one in Universal Consciousness. Everything we perceive stems from the same source.

But don't just take my word for this. I would encourage you to examine all the facts you can regarding the nature of reality for yourself, adding in your own experiences, and not accepting the consensus of your Belief

System. This examination will enable you to see for yourself whether reality is an illusion.

Why The Inconvenient Joke is so Inconvenient

Aside from making many jobs obsolete and detrimental to our economy, another untold, unconscious reason for our refusal to laugh at the Cosmic Joke is because we have an enormous stake in the "reality" of the Illusory World. Think about it - everything we have done since around the time of our birth has enhanced our belief in this illusion. If we were to suddenly begin to laugh at it, we would essentially be laughing at almost everything we have done and believed our entire life.

Cognitive dissonance causes it to be very inconvenient to laugh at The Joke. Cognitive dissonance results in psychological stress in a person who simultaneously holds two contradictory **beliefs, regardless of how valid those beliefs may be.** When confronted with new information that contradicts engrained and conditioned false beliefs, cognitive dissonance causes us to avoid the psychological stress that will result from accepting these new beliefs. Even though we may know the old belief is false, that our world is real and that we are separate entities, we hold onto this belief because it is convenient.

The good news is that cognitive dissonance requires thoughts. A way of resolving the psychological stresses that result from cognitive dissonance is to laugh at our thoughts.

But the challenge of laughing away our thoughts goes even deeper. This is because most of us derive our complete identity through our thoughts. Think about this for a moment: If you were not able to identify yourself through word-based thoughts, who would you be?

Giving up thoughts really means giving up our sense of self. This can be extremely frightening! This is why I experienced tears during my Vipassana meditation when I felt like I died when I had no thoughts. This is an unconscious reason we have difficulty laughing at The Joke and at our thoughts, and why we may make every excuse not to laugh. The mind and the ego are battling for their survival by keeping The Joke completely hidden, even though it is now completely exposed.

Another reason why laughing at The Inconvenient Joke can be so inconvenient is because it means taking 100% responsibility for all our reflections in our Hall of Mirrors, including those we may despise. Although even the suggestion of this may seem overwhelmingly repugnant and may cause you an intense desire to burn this book, it can be the most empowering thing we can do.

Although there might be people all around us who seem to be causing us to suffer, once we take 100% responsibility for our reflections, we will see this "response-ability" as our ability-to-respond in a powerful way, an opportunity to see the distortions that need cleaning.

Taking 100% responsibility will result in having what psychologists call an extremely high "Internal Locus of Control." People who have a very high Internal Locus of Control believe that they control their destiny. According to a June 30, 2011 issue of Psychology Today, psychologists have found that the number one contributor to happiness is not money nor good looks nor popularity nor a hot sex life, but having a high Internal Locus of Control.

A nationwide survey conducted by the University of Michigan reported that the 15% of Americans who have a high Internal Locus of Control also raved about having "extraordinarily positive feelings of happiness."

Since we may never know the true nature of reality with absolute certainty, doesn't it seem wise to believe in one that can bring "extraordinarily positive feelings of happiness" and empowerment, especially when there is a solid scientific basis for it?

To do this in the most powerful way in which we regain our Wholeness and reconnect with our God essence, we need to take 100% responsibility for all our reflections.

This may have been how Jesus was able to perform miracles. When Jesus said, "I and the Father are one," He likely meant that He was perfectly aligned with the light and power of God.

Jesus also said, "Very truly I tell you, whoever believes in me will do the works I have been doing, and they will do even greater things than these because I am going to the Father." This suggests that we can perform greater miracles than Jesus did by following in His footsteps. But how is this possible?

Being able to say "I and the Father are one" is the key to miracles. **Even though only Jesus said, "I and the Father are one," in our non-local reality in which everyone and everything is interconnected, is it possible that I and the Father can ever be separate? Is it possible that we are all one with the Father?**

Although it takes a great deal of courage to take 100% responsibility for all our reflections, to embrace our interconnectedness, and to laugh at the Inconvenient Joke, this may be what is required to experience miracles and help heal our world.

How to Live as "Spiritual Beings Having a Human Experience"

While many of us believe we are "spiritual beings having a human experience," we are so associated into our bodies that we often behave as though we are human beings having a spiritual experience. This strong association with our body creates an attachment to it and can lead to a great deal of suffering.

This is what I experienced during my Vipassana meditation when I was completely associated with my body and experienced excruciating pain. Once I witnessed myself dissociated from my body by watching myself from the ceiling, the pain was completely eradicated.

Laughing at The Joke can accomplish a similar dissociation. Wholeheartedly Laughing at The Cosmic Joke can enable us to dissociate with the suffering associated with human experience and help enable us to enjoy the process of living as Spiritual Beings having a human experience.

Laughter: The Rational Response to a Reality That's Not Real

An essential component of laughter is called the "surprise of the discovery." A joke leads us one way, and then suddenly shifts our perceptions at the punchline. An example of this is the Groucho Marx joke, "Yesterday I fed an elephant in my pajamas. How it got in my pajamas, I have no idea."

The funniest jokes invoke the highest intensity of sensory modalities and the greatest surprise. Generally, the more serious the set-up to the punchline, the better the laughter.

Often, the longer the suspense of the set-up, the greater the surprise and the greater the laughter. Many joke set-ups occur within one, two, or several sentences; some go on even longer with elaborate details that help build the suspense. The set-up for the Inconvenient Joke often has a long build-up of suspense, is very visual, very serious, uses the vast intensity of all our sensory modalities, and has been taking place throughout our life.

If the set-up of several sentences can bring about such intense laughter, imagine the intensity of the laughter once you laugh at the grand punchline of the Inconvenient Joke. Its set-up involved *all* your senses and has been occurring throughout the many years of your "life sentence" of believing you were a victim of your reflections. When the surprise of the discovery finally happens, the eruption of an entire lifetime of built-up laughter can be enormous. For these reasons, the Inconvenient Joke is the Most Powerful Joke ever told.

Once we truly take the time to fully grasp the ramifications of core teachings of quantum physicists, religions and spiritual teachers, we will have no rational response other than laughter.

Once we fully let go of all the barriers, this laughter may erupt intensively at what some may consider being the best Joke ever told. During a Holotropic Breathwork workshop I attended several years ago, I laughed hysterically at The Joke for about 2 ½ hours. From this experience, I found that Laughing at the Inconvenient Joke has the potential of changing a "life sentence" of suffering into a life sentence of how to structure our thoughts consisting of 11 words – "As soon as you have made a thought, laugh at it!"

In the remainder of this book, we will discuss The Joke is greater detail and ways of eradicating blockages to laughter. It is essential to eliminate these blockages because if we are not laughing at the Cosmic Joke, we are predisposed to suffering from an Illusion of Hell that we don't even recognize.

What is the solution to eradicating blockages to our authentic laughter?

The *solution* is dis-*solution* of illusion-based thoughts.

"Just as true humor is laughter at oneself,
true humanity is knowledge of oneself."
— Alan Watts

Chapter Eight
Dissolving Negative Emotions

Although we often do everything possible to eliminate negative emotions, when we really think about it, negative emotions can be beneficial. They often serve as a test to make sure we are laughing at the Inconvenient Joke. When we are taking the world too seriously and have taken a bit of a snooze from laughing at The Joke, our negative emotions can serve as tickle-alarms that test us.

Regardless of gender, we all have ***test-tickles*** - negative emotions arising from our Frankenstein Monsters that test us and tickle us awake to make sure we are laughing at the Jokes.

Test-tickles are all around us. The puns which are strategically sprinkled throughout this book are your test-tickles. They are there to make sure you are not taking this book too seriously, and because one path to enlightenment is to lighten up.

It may seem completely reasonable for someone to have negative emotions if they have cancer, chronic pain and other health challenges, or are behind on their mortgage payments or with a partner who is verbally and physically abusive. It may seem irrational to expect people who are suffering to laugh at the Inconvenient Joke, even if that laughter might help heal their circumstances.

In fact, laughter may not be appropriate for everyone. Sometimes when we get a bit behind in laughing at our thoughts and at the Inconvenient Joke, things can get overwhelming. This is why the underlined words of Lao Tzu's teaching are so important – "**As soon as** you have made a thought, laugh at it." Laughing at each thought as soon as it arises is like taking our daily vitamins and eating our fruits and vegetables. It's like cleaning each dish instead of waiting for a mountain of dirty dishes to pile up. The longer thoughts fester in the mind, the more destruction they can cause.

One may wonder how it would be possible to function in our daily life without thoughts. How can we do our work or have a normal conversation with our friends and family?

We do this by laughing away our robotic, culturally conditioned, habitual thoughts, and engaging in our daily activities from a space beyond those thoughts. We do this from a space in which we have completely surrendered, yet are empowered and animated. From this space, we are being walked and talked by God/Higher Power, as we act from The Zone - a space in which there is no volitional doing or speaking.

Laughing as soon as we've made a thought is a fun way to surrender to God's Higher Power. Waiting for overwhelming life challenges to remind us to laugh is another option to surrender. I choose the first of these options.

Regardless of which option we prefer, we can always choose to laugh at our thoughts about our situation for the reasons listed in chapter six.

But laughter is not for everyone at every time. Rules are made to be broken - when breaking those rules is truly justified. In some cases, it may be fine to fully embrace and release the emotions that arise from our overwhelming challenges - just as a child throws a tantrum when he is full of rage. Half an hour later, she is playing with her friends in the playground, having forgotten completely what happened earlier.

Since negative emotions are tickling us to laugh at our thoughts, let's see how this happens with specific emotions:

- **Anger** always seems justified by our thoughts. Many people are addicted to anger because, after many years of holding onto it, it feels like a part of them. Some people would feel out of balance without anger. Although they may say they want to feel peace, unconsciously they choose their old friend.

Once we bring this unconsciousness to conscious awareness and see how anger has affected us, we are in a position of choice and power. Once we are in this place of power, we have many options. These include doing nothing or throwing a cathartic tantrum until we have expressed all our anger and rage.

After we have completely expressed our outrage, we can laugh at the Inconvenient Joke, laugh at our thoughts, or undergo **_LaughGnosis_** to help us laugh at our thoughts and the Cosmic Joke more easily.

Once we can laugh at our thoughts, the negative emotion becomes a call to take empowered action, such as making sure we know all we can about the best cancer and chronic pain treatment and following up with our doctor as necessary.

By choosing to let go of our anger in this way, we are choosing to exchange it for the ability to take more empowered and effective action from The Zone.

- **Fear** is the belief that the distortions in the lens can somehow harm our **_true Self._** Instead of cleaning the distortions in our lens by realizing that within the non-local reality in which we live there is nothing to fear, we are mesmerized by our fearful projections.

  Like anger, fear also seems justified by our thoughts when we forget to laugh at them. Fear can be very helpful to trigger our fight or flight response when we need to run away from a saber-toothed tiger. Until such time that we are able to completely clean our lens, such fear is entirely rational. The problem is that many people are stuck in this response and do nothing to help clear their lens. Chronic fear can result in fatigue due to adrenal gland burn-out. The need for coffee and/or sugar in order to be functional squeezes any remaining adrenal reserve.

  People experiencing fatigue are sometimes treated with Adderall, which squeezes and drains the adrenals even more. The problem is, without this medication, these unfortunate people are often incapacitated because instead of being treated for an Adderall deficiency, they should have been treated for a laughter deficiency. By using laughter as their medicine, they would have all the biochemical benefits of their own powerful neurotransmitters and could see their fearful situation from a clearer perspective. **Laughter is like taking very potent, natural, uncontrolled, legal, free drugs.**

- <u>Grief</u> is the anguish that a person may experience after a significant loss, such as the death of a beloved. Although very profound grief may be felt for their reflection in your grand Hall of Mirrors, the part of you that created that reflection is always with you. This part of you may create a different reflection, such as the person's spirit being with you wherever you go. Cleansing tears based on the "perceived" separation from our loved ones is completely normal. Eventually we will see the situation from The Zone, that God Space in which everyone is always inter-connected at the deepest level, even after death. When we do, we may eventually laugh at the Inconvenient Joke that, within our interconnected non-local reality, separation from anything is impossible.

One of the best characteristics of laughter is that it is alchemy for emotions. Fear and grief are among the lowest levels of emotions. Love, joy, freedom, appreciation, and gratitude are among the highest. Once we understand God's sense of humor, we can laugh at life's challenges. This will enable us to transform fear or grief into love, joy, freedom or gratitude. This form of alchemy can save years of therapy.

- <u>Worry</u> is another common emotion that can pull our thoughts out of The Zone. Worry is the concern that the images reflected in the mirrors may pose an unexpected threat. We give our power away to our reflections instead of laughing at them. Once we laugh at how silly it is to worry about our reflections, we are grateful to those reflections for alerting us to the distortions on our lens which created them. This process takes us to gratitude, laughter, and joy, which as we will see later, are the highest vibrational levels of emotions.

Worry can be an effective way to turn our attention to planning actions to change something that is within our capacity to change. The challenge is that worry and planning can take us out of the present moment - the only moment in which we can access The Zone. The way to plan for the future yet stay in the present moment is by staying completely focused on each aspect of the plan at every moment, and being utterly unattached to the result.

We are often reluctant to give up worry because it seems to give us useful information. The problem is that sometimes we worry about things over which we have no control and situations in which all the worrying in the world will not change anything. Nevertheless, worrying can be very helpful when practiced effectively.

How to Worry Effectively

In order to worry effectively, I recommend that people make a list of at least 50 things to worry intensively about for one hour.

Please begin sentences with "What if... (i.e. What if the world explodes tomorrow afternoon?)"

Never use sentences that begin with, "How can I?" or "What would it take?"

If you can't take an hour to worry, please add that to your worry list.

On the worry list, please write only things over which you seem to have absolutely no control. Things like the weather, the war in the Middle East, and your less than perfect childhood.

Then, please begin a second worry list. On this second list, write all the things you may be able to control, like your thoughts about any of the above. Items in this list are not included in the 50 items on the first worry list.

If you have difficulty coming up with 50 things to worry about, some tips are – the on-going tensions in the Middle East, global warming is getting worse, and more seals in Japan are dying every day.

If you still cannot come up with a list of 50 items, start worrying about this as well, and add that to your first worry list.

If you don't have at least 50 items on your list, please list things you forgot to worry about in the past or things you will likely need to worry about 20 years from now.

Limit your intensive worry sessions to just worrying. Please refrain from problem-solving during this hour.

If you think about something to worry about after that hour, write it down as part of your worry list for the next day.

If you worry about something outside the hour allotted, please worry about it during a set time for at least 15 minutes the following day.

No problem solving is allowed for the first three days. After those three days, one hour per day of problem solving is permitted.

After this exercise, most people realize that there are many things over which they have no control. Although they may have plenty of troubles, most of their worries have never happened and never will.

Changing Our Ideas about What Requires Change

We often find that when we are no longer able to change a situation, the challenge is to change ourselves. Rumi said, "**Yesterday I was clever, so I wanted to change the world. Today I am wise, so I am changing myself.**" One way we change ourselves is by changing our thoughts and beliefs about our situation by laughing at our thoughts.

Viktor Frankl, the creator of *Logotherapy,* found that people in concentration camps realized that everything can be taken away from someone except one thing - the freedom to choose one's attitude about any situation. There were prisoners in the concentration camps who suffered intense emotional anguish. Others used their freedom to choose their emotions in a positive way. When we use this freedom, no person or situation will ever have the remote-control button to our emotions again.

Most of the time, we become so intensely identified with our thoughts and mesmerized by the world of illusion that we forget to laugh at the Cosmic Joke. By laughing at the Cosmic Joke, we use our mind to get us beyond our mind. It helps us escape our Illusory World.

The fact is, the harder we try to escape The Illusion, the more we will be its slave. Trying hard to escape The Illusion takes us out of alignment with accepting "what is" and creates more distortions on our lens.

I want to make it very clear that our Illusory World is not our enemy. Because it shows us our blockages to wholeness by revealing our distortions that need healing, it is our greatest gift. Only by our persistent laughter at the Joke will this Hellish illusion be transcended.

Whenever we laugh at the Inconvenient Joke and at our thoughts, we are realigning with the light and power of God. Our continued laughter at The Joke and at our thoughts helps dissolve the thoughts that created the distortions in our lens.

We cannot escape the Illusion of Hell through strenuous efforts, but we *can* laugh our way out. Every time we laugh at the Powerful Joke and at our thoughts, we are dissolving another distortion on our lens. This process may go on for quite some time until there are no distortions. At that time, we will experience perfect peace and the Heavenly appearance of the Light of God reflecting right back to us.

Whenever we experience any other negative emotion, we are sinning against ourselves and setting off irritations that are also our tickle alarms. They are alerting us to distortions on our lens that may require laughter to clear.

It is humbling to realize that whenever we have any negative emotion or think of ourselves as anything less than magnificent, we are committing a sin against ourselves.

Although it would be ideal to think of ourselves as perfect, I admittedly feel like I have more flaws than the Empire State Building, as can sometimes be seen in my not-so-funny puns.

To give you an idea of how bad my puns are, I once entered a local paper's pun contest. I sent in ten different puns, in the hope that at least one of the puns would win. Unfortunately, no-pun-in-ten-did.

Fortunately, it is not necessary to laugh at my puns, but it is necessary to wake up laughing at the Inconvenient Joke.

Every time we laugh at the Inconvenient Joke, we are taking another step away from being mesmerized by our hall of Frankenstein Monsters and are diffusing any related negative emotions. All negative emotions are the result of a laughter deficiency.

All the Frankenstein Monsters in our life are putting in an award-winning performance by showing us our blockages to living a life outside the Illusory World. Once we see how we are creating these reflections in our Hall of Mirrors, we can then clear the distortions on our lens. This will allow us to align with the Light of God by laughing at the Inconvenient Joke. We will then live in The Zone and see the miracles of God reflected back to us in our Hall of Mirrors.

Until we can fully comprehend the literally earth-shattering ramifications of the Powerful Joke and laugh at it wholeheartedly, we can still use laughter constructively as a weapon of mass destruction against our fixed beliefs.

"Life cannot be against you for you are life itself."
— Mooji

Chapter Nine
Weapons of Mass Distraction

It may be challenging to envision living a life beyond the Illusory World – a life lived in a state of profound inner peace and Bliss – while appearing to live in a world full of chaos, mass distractions, and weapons of mass destruction.

This is because, although numerous Nobel Laureates repeatedly say this world is an illusion, we are so mesmerized by this Illusory World held together by thought, that we lose the plot.

We see the weapons of mass destruction and overlook the most destructive weapon of all - our restless "monkey mind." One of the greatest annihilation experts who ever lived was neither Mr. Adolph Hitler nor Mr. Jozef Stalin, but "Mr. Monkey Mind." Allowing our "monkey mind" to make our decisions is like putting Jack Daniels in the driver's seat and going on a wild ride. That's a whole different way of being driven by the holy "spirit."

To make this picture seem more frightening, we have world leaders with access to the nuclear codes who have monkey minds; they sometimes seem like Jack Daniels on steroids.

In the past, despite going to countless workshops on unconditional love, I became overwhelmingly enraged by the behavior of some world leaders. I took my Frankenstein Monsters to be very real.

The fact that others were also brainwashed by their dualistic thinking to be enraged by their reflection was of no consolation. After all, the consensus reality of everyone in a dream is that the dream characters are real.

This dualistic brainwashing had hijacked my mind to become my biggest weapon of mass destruction. It was on a collision course with our

True, non-dualistic reality - a course that is guaranteed to cause total annihilation.

The weapons of mass destruction that we were led to believe existed in Iraq and the hijacked planes that hit the World Trade Center were all a product of this mind-based weapon. The devastation resulting from the hijacking of those planes does not compare with the destruction resulting from allowing our thoughts to be hijacked by our dualistic thinking of believing there is anything that is separate from us within our interconnected, non-dualistic, reality.

The Greatest Terrorist That Ever Lived is Closer than You Think

Based on my experiences and research, we have massively more effect on the so-called outer world than we know. The world we see is merely a projection of our thoughts; therefore the terrorists and the Frankenstein Monsters in our life are a projection of the fears and anger in our own mind. Terrorists are merely a product of a distortion in our lens – a distortion resulting from our belief in separation. This belief in separation, resulting in dualistic thinking, is the main unlaughed at Joke. It is the cause of all suffering that has ever existed because it creates the illusion that something outside of us can terrorize Who We Really Are.

Our minds are constantly being distracted by the fear-provoking "*daily news.*" This daily news is actually a "*daily noose*" around our neck – it is one of our "**weapons of mass distraction.**"

It may seem as though the most challenging people and situations in our life are our most significant weapons of mass destruction and the causes of suffering. It may seem as though the guilty person is a family member, a politician, or the evil people in the world. It may also be convenient to blame the media for hijacking our thoughts. But since our thoughts create our reality, **it is less dangerous to allow planes to be hijacked and "terrorize" tall buildings than to allow our minds to be hijacked.** A hijacked mind can potentially terrorize not only every tall building but our entire lives and everything else we believe to be real.

107

Our life is like a murder mystery in which the guilty party becomes more and more apparent. The guilty person in many murder mysteries is often someone like a butler – the person who is least suspected but is always at the scene of the crime.

As we think back to our most challenging life situations, we may realize that there was always one common denominator - our thoughts. Like the butler, our thoughts are the least-suspected party, but always present at all the scenes in our life. Our thoughts are sinful because, as we know from our definition of sin, they take us out of alignment with the light and power of God.

The culprits are not only thoughts that result in fear, worry, grief or judgment of ourselves or others, but all thoughts that have not yet been sufficiently laughed at and remain as obstacles to our entry into The Zone. There are no neutral thoughts. An "idle thought" is an oxymoron. All thinking produces form at some level. We may have believed that our thoughts are pure, innocent and ineffectual, just playing in the "background." Who would have believed that they were the biggest problem all along? Even though the "Victimizers" in our life clearly seem to be the guilty parties, that label really belongs only to our thoughts, the most dangerous Frankenstein Monsters of them all.

During my ten-day meditation retreat, experimenting internally with the relationship between pain, bliss, and mindlessness, I found that thoughts alone had prevented me from experiencing profound Bliss. Even the thought of Bliss interfered with the experience of it.

When we are willing and able to laugh at our thoughts, we realize that we are not our thoughts. Until this becomes clear, there may be a tendency to feel depressed when having depressing thoughts and happy when having happy thoughts. This tendency puts us on a constant roller coaster of thoughts and emotions that can spin us around and make us sick.

This roller coaster ride may continue until we finally realize that - unlike our mind that changes from moment to moment - Who We Really Are, underneath the ride, does not change. With this realization, we can sit back and watch our thoughts go on the wildest ride they like, and enjoy this entertainment.

If we negatively judge our mind, we risk its revenge. Instead, it is more useful to appreciate our mind for all the help it gives us and retrain it to help us even more.

We retrain our mind by teaching it to laugh at the Inconvenient Joke and at our thoughts. When we laugh at the Inconvenient Joke, we are using our biggest weapon of mass *destruction* on our weapon of mass *distraction*. Instead of seeking its destruction, we are helping the mind to laugh, which helps us to transcend the mind.

We do that by stepping back and watching the monkey mind from a place of amusement, one step closer to the exit door from the Illusory World. The thoughts we took so seriously for all those years, we now listen to as entertainment. We notice how hard it's trying to get our attention, making louder and louder noises in the monkey mind version of guerrilla warfare. In the meantime, we laugh with amusement at all this monkey business, realizing that a monkey is just a "chimp off the old block."

For many years, we derived our whole identity from these chimps. Now we can watch them with amusement and see that neither their behavior nor their bananas have "a-ppeal.".

"Those who talk don't know.
Those who know don't talk... *they laugh."*
— Lao Tzu... (with *words in Italic by Mitchell J. Bloom, M.D.*)

Chapter Ten
Thought Addicts Anonymous

By now you may agree that laughter is good medicine. At the same time, you may have also realized that laughing at the Inconvenient Joke and/or at our thoughts – even though it sounds so easy, so powerful and so much fun – can seem more challenging than asking a politician to stop lying.

Just as lying politicians are not anonymous, thought addicts are not anonymous either. They are just so much more common; they seem normal.

Letting go of conditioned thoughts is so vitally important to our ability to live our life in The Zone, with a deep sense of inner peace and Bliss. Not letting them go keeps us from laughing at the Inconvenient Joke. Let's take more time to examine the perceived power of thought. Doing so can help dissolve its power and help unleash our Laughter. Let's also discuss ways of dissolving some specific conditioned thoughts that create barriers to our Authentic Laughter.

But first I must admit - I have essentially been the highly disheveled guy with track marks in every vein, shooting up thought after thought in a back alley, addicted to the most powerful drugs of all, personally delivered by my junkie, the Monkey Mind. I was using them on a daily basis since early childhood – as was the rest of humanity.

A Course in Miracles says, "Every thought you have makes up some segment of the world you see[1]." With every thought, we are essentially shooting up another vein and are creating another part of our wild hallucination we call our world. But even though we are shooting these powerful hallucinogens into our vein, rest assured....it's not all in "vain." It is presenting us with a fascinating opportunity to see how our thoughts influence our experiences of the world at a very visceral level - creating a virtual trip through Hell.

Perhaps you believe, like I did, that the world is not a Hell at all, but that it is a Utopia. But once I experienced a mind free of thoughts and the bliss of seeing beyond thoughts during my Vipassana meditation, I realized how naïve I had been.

Most of us will admit that we have a vice and/or an addiction, whether it is chocolate, smoking, coffee, etc., but we look at that vice as the problem. Once we look deeper, we may discover something more profound. These vices, and indeed all our suffering, are the product of the worst addiction of all – our usual forms of thinking.

According to the American Society of Addiction Medicine, an addiction "is characterized by an inability to consistently abstain, impairment in behavioral control, craving, diminished recognition of significant problems with one's behaviors and interpersonal relationships, and a dysfunctional emotional response."

Thoughts fit this definition better than anything else classified as an addiction, probably better than heroin and cocaine combined. Cocaine has a very short half-life for a drug, so withdrawal symptoms can begin as soon as 90 minutes after the last dose. Heroin withdrawal symptoms start within 6-12 hours of the previous dose. But observe what happens if most people try to go without thoughts for even one minute.

Thoughts are indeed the invisible drivers of many vices and addictions and often go untreated.

"Thoughtism" is totally unrecognized, yet much more deadly than alcoholism. In addition to AA and NA groups, there is a definite need for TA support groups. Thought Addiction Anonymous groups could have a similar twelve step program for addiction to thoughts as AA does for addiction to alcohol. The only requirement for Thoughts Anonymous membership is a desire to begin laughing at the Inconvenient Joke and at one's thoughts, whatever they may be.

The main advantage of alcoholism over "thoughtism" is that alcoholics are aware of a problem and are therefore easier to treat. In fact, "thoughtism" can be a leading cause of drug and alcohol addictions.

Unlike cocaine, which people know is not normal to use, "thoughtism" is considered normal. Everyone is highly addicted, and we are allowing this addiction to run our lives, and the lives of everyone around us, every moment of every day.

That is not to say we need to abstain entirely from all thoughts, or that some thoughts are not necessary or helpful. The problem is in being mesmerized by our thoughts and allowing them to hijack us from The Zone.

Once we continue laughing at our conditioned thoughts, spontaneous thoughts that are more aligned with being in The Zone will emerge. As we continue this process, laughing will become more natural and spontaneous and will enable us to get progressively deeper into The Zone.

The Deadliest Vice of All

Let's face it, most of us have many vices and bad habits. As dangerous as those known vices may be, the deadliest of all may be the one of which many of us are unaware. This stealth vice causes our identification with our body resulting in our fear of death - the mother of most fears and the underlying cause of many negative emotions and addictions.

Our addictions provide us with fleeting imitations of a fullness that can only truly be fulfilled by letting go of our addictions and facing the Abyss of having no thoughts.

When we boil down most vices and addictions, we are left with thoughts. Thoughts create our beliefs regarding what helps us relax and what we need to do to cope with stress, as well as what makes us look cool and what constitutes an excuse for a break. Thoughts also contribute to the addictive properties of substances.

Our thoughts convince us that cigarettes are highly addictive, but is this true? How many times have smokers slept eight hours without craving a cigarette when they thought they were addicted to smoking every few hours? If they were as addicted as they thought, they would be waking up every few hours craving a cigarette.

While we overestimate the addictive properties of cigarettes, our society unknowingly tries to underestimate the addictive properties of conditioned thoughts.

We spend our whole life trying to fill a deep emptiness in our heart, in our stomach, and in our soul, which can only be genuinely filled directly by God – the Divine Nature behind our conditioned thoughts. Instead of opening to this emptiness, we create vices and addictions which we use as protection from facing our Abyss. These vices are but a mere taste of what we can experience once we've faced our Abyss. We will talk more about this process of facing the Abyss in chapter 14.

Instead of facing this Abyss, we shoot up with yet another thought in this never-ending global acid trip from Hell. But because everyone is taking the same potent dose, we call it normal. We are oblivious of what we are doing and remember not to laugh at how well we convince ourselves this Global acid trip from Hell is normal.

By now we know that the way of breaking this addiction to the thoughts that are creating this illusion is by laughing at the Powerful Joke. However, we are so addicted to the Illusory World that we may still find it difficult to laugh. Until we are ready to let go of our addiction to our conditioned thoughts and are able to laugh at the Inconvenient Joke, forgiveness is very helpful.

"The weak can never forgive. Forgiveness is the attribute of the strong."
— Mahatma Gandhi

Chapter Eleven
The "F" Word

In our journey to find our authentic laughter, it is helpful to find the most dangerous thoughts interfering with it. These most dangerous thoughts are those resulting from resistance to forgiveness and unconditional love. Hence, the best ways to unleash this laughter are through forgiveness and unconditional love.

Our ego is responsible for all the distortions on our lens. Forgiveness, because it is the most frightening word to the ego, is the naughtiest "F" word of all. It is the "F" word we can use to screw the ego right out of a job.

Still, the ego is not the enemy. We have somehow learned that in this whole spiritual game of cops and robbers, the ego is the robber that needs to be killed. But this is not the case. It is doing its job perfectly. Our job is not to be free of our ego, for that is virtually impossible. Resisting the ego will only make it stronger. Helping it to help us is the best option.

Our ego wants the best for us. It is trying to help us be happy in the way it knows best. Rather than trying to get rid of it, it may be better to re-educate it in a way that is helpful to both us and our ego.

As you recall, the ego is the part that gives us the feeling of individuality and craving for material possessions. It creates the illusion of separation because it believes that this is the best way for us to be safe. It is through forgiveness that the "disease of the ego".......does-ease-and-go. Once our ego realizes that laughing at the Inconvenient Joke can bring both of us even more happiness, our ego can help in this process.

Instead of being angry at our ego for making it seem so hard to find forgiveness, it is best to laugh at our thoughts alongside the ego - so that

114

we can both be happy. This allows the ego to drop its old agenda and take on this new one – the laughter agenda. But until we can wholeheartedly laugh at the Joke and our thoughts alongside the ego, forgiveness can be extremely helpful.

Although there may be many evil people in the world who may not seem worthy of forgiveness, it is not up to us to change anyone. Within our interconnected reality, "others" are merely acting out their roles of bringing to our attention the parts of our mind that need to be healed.

The Benefit of "F"ing Someone

If we were abused by a relative, it is tempting to carry that anger around with us for the rest of our life. It is also possible to pass on that anger to our children and to generations to come.

Instead of holding onto that anger, we may want to consider whether our relative is merely acting out their role - to bring to our attention the parts of our subconscious mind that are blocking our experience of Wholeness. "In a sense," forgiveness allows us to see their "innocence." Once we heal this anger blockage internally through forgiveness, the outer blame game is over – for us, our children, and generations to come.

If we no longer experience dishonest and abusive people, it may seem difficult to find politicians. But as we evolve through forgiveness, so will our politicians, because they are merely a reflection of our mind. Since objective reality is a gigantic hologram, as our portion of the hologram changes, so does every other part, including politicians.

If we continue to hold on to anger and political division, the holographic reflections we perceive as our politicians may give us more to get divided and angry about. But as we realize that these politicians are gifts reflected back to our attention for healing through forgiveness, we will begin to see our old anger as a bunch of poppycock, and a better world can begin to manifest for all.

There are many ways of forgiving others. We could write a letter letting a world leader know we forgive them for bringing about our economic collapse by selling out to the global bankers. We could forgive them for their perceived role in the killing of millions of people in ludicrous wars whose goal was to make money for the military industrial complex.

Whether we write a letter or speak to the person directly doesn't matter as much as really feeling True forgiveness for them from the bottom of our heart.

I have done several hypnosis sessions in which I worked with my anger toward politicians. A great benefit of hypnosis is that I was able to step into the other person's shoes to swap roles and see the situation from their perspective, given their conditioned belief system and early childhood experiences. Through this process, I felt more of what they feel and was able to gain a better understanding of the situation. From this more holistic perspective, I was in a much better position to forgive.

This process may be more effective in a hypnotic state than talking with the person face to face, because when in that hypnotic state, we can have a 360-degree perspective outside of our usual mental construct walls. From this expanded perspective, forgiveness may come much easier.

I have also undergone past life regressions where I was able to see the grand karmic dance in which I kept switching from victim to Victimizer for generations after generations, as far back as I could go. I gained a great appreciation for how victimization and the need for revenge can go on forever. It was carried with me lifetime after lifetime because this instinct was so embedded into my subconscious mind.

Based on the anger and victimization karmic dance I had been playing, that pattern could have continued for many lifetimes. But once I forgave my Frankenstein Monsters - after seeing the situation from their perspective - the tide turned. Forgiveness washed away that karma, and the game was over!

More importantly, I thanked my "Victimizers" for being my greatest teachers by helping me see my biggest obstacle to having a clear lens. After forgiving them, I felt much more peaceful, whole and complete.

There are many levels of forgiveness. To someone entirely new to the power of forgiveness, I offer them the "Ten Steps to Forgiveness."

Ten Steps to Forgiveness

To help you heal and find the peace that comes from forgiveness, you can take the following steps:

1. Allow yourself to fully accept, welcome, and observe yourself experiencing the anger.

2. Realize that anger is a choice. You can hold onto anger, or set yourself free from it.

3. Ask yourself what you truly want. Do you want anger and all its adverse health consequences, or would you prefer to take a DIP into Deep Inner Peace?

4. Understand that forgiveness does not condone nor forget the harmful acts. You forgive the doer, not what was done.

5. Realize that you are responsible for your own feelings, and for healing the hurt that is going on inside you. Understand that if you allow yourself to get dragged into anger, you're giving your power away to the very person you resent.

6. Take full responsibility for your part in whatever happened, understanding that things happen for a reason. Do this without blame or guilt. See the situation as an opportunity for healing and growth. Try to identify the part of you that may have attracted this situation in order to learn a big life lesson or to burn some karma from this or a previous lifetime.

7. Decide to forgive, even if this decision is half-hearted at first. This will probably reduce your general anxiety immediately. Notice any blocks or barriers that present themselves.

8. Notice whether the need to feel like a victim or the need to be right and make the other person wrong comes up. Is this what you really want, or is physical and emotional health, happiness and Deep Inner Peace what you seek?

9. Realize that forgiving is a courageous act. It is a present that you give yourself. It has nothing to do with whether the other person can admit that they are wrong.

10. Remember that you are determined to find the pure joy and Deep Inner Peace that true forgiveness can bring to your life. Be willing to learn and do whatever it takes to forgive.

The important thing to realize is that since we live in a non-local reality in which separation is an illusion, there is no one outside of you. Therefore, there is no one you need to forgive other than yourself for believing in separation.

Although forgiveness is extremely helpful and is the primary teaching of many spiritual practices, it still keeps us focused on the mind, and on the Illusory World created by thoughts. The need for forgiveness is a good step but is nonetheless a product of thought. The presence of thought is what keeps us mesmerized by The Illusion.

Without thought, there is no need for forgiveness. Therefore, **Powerful Laughter at thoughts can be even more powerful than forgiveness**, because it releases all need for forgiveness and liberates us from the Illusory World. But until we are willing and able to laugh at the Joke and at our thoughts, forgiveness is helpful.

"Darkness cannot drive out darkness; only light can do that.
Hate cannot drive out hate; only love can do that."
— Martin Luther King, Jr.

Chapter Twelve
Unconditional Love Meets Adolph Hitler

There is another effective cleaning fluid for our lens – it is unconditional love. Combining forgiveness with unconditional love enhances our ability to laugh at the Powerful Joke by loosening our attachment to our perceived divisions within the Illusory World.

Some emotional and health challenges can result from distortions on our lens resulting from those we have not yet forgiven and do not unconditionally love. To make sure our mirror is as clear as possible, it is helpful to ask ourselves a simple question - Is there anyone you still have difficulty unconditionally loving?

If you believe you love everyone unconditionally, you may then ask yourself if you forgive and unconditionally love Adolph Hitler.

Although that question may seem absurd, any resistance to forgiveness and unconditional love implies some degree of judgment about all the Hitlers in our world - those people it seems impossible to forgive and love. Yes, I am talking about the one that just popped into your mind, the one you thought I couldn't possibly mean. No, I'm not kidding, and I'm sorry if I am slowly turning into one of your Hitlers by suggesting you do something this seemingly "impossible." You are free to rip up this book, burn it, call me every expletive imaginable and give this book atrocious reviews if that makes you happy, but what will that accomplish? Your judgment of all your Hitlers causes toxins in your body which can cause disease. Instead of judging these Hitlers, a more helpful way to see their actions is by laughing at your judgmental thoughts until you reach discernment.

The difference between judgment and discernment is that judgment is a condescending, emotionally charged action that introduces resistance and polarization. It encourages separation between ourselves and the one we judge. Judgment also generates harmful biochemistry in the body, which can eventually cause disease.

The subconscious voice behind judgment is different from the voice behind discernment. The subconscious voice that is running a judgmental reaction would sound something like this: "that raving lunatic is so dreadful that I need to go into fight or flight mode to be safe. I'll risk giving myself a stroke or heart attack to show that idiot how wrong he is and how broken-hearted and angry I am."

Discernment, on the other hand, is a non-judgmental way of seeing things as they are. This way of seeing is not a product of rigid standards, opinions, or social pressures. Discernment often comes from laughing at our judgmental thoughts. It allows us to make empowered choices rather than disempowered and reactionary ones.

Discernment is not emotionally charged and does not introduce a feeling of separation. It is also much healthier for the body. It allows us to find the God essence that is in everyone but may seem buried deeply beneath their actions. This God essence is naturally lovable in anyone and everyone.

The subconscious voice behind moving from judgment to discernment can be, "I wonder how I will see this person or situation, and how much more empowered I will feel, after I laugh away my judgmental thoughts."

Laughing at **_God's Jokes_** converts judgment into discernment and helps eliminate its emotional charge. It also helps remove the distortions on our lens caused by anger. It allows us to love the other person, even though we may wholeheartedly disagree with their actions.

By changing judgment into discernment, this laughter changes Disempowered Resistance into Empowered Peace and Love. It also allows our actions to flow from The Zone - the place of Absolute Power. Although the actions we take from judgment and discernment may look exactly the same on the outside, they are dramatically different on the inside. This makes all the difference in the world and occurs because whatever is in our internal world reflects back to us in the mirrors of the external world. Empowered and loving emotions result in empowered and loving reflections.

Once we see all the Hitlers in our life through discerning and unconditionally loving eyes, we may be able to see the God Essence within them. This often sounds much easier than it is but should be much easier by the end of this chapter.

Although it may seem repulsive, this means Unconditionally Loving all your Hitlers. If you find it difficult to do right now, please skip to the next section. If you feel courageous and would like to take a giant leap into The Zone, let's plunge into Love.

What is Love?

For starters, let's define love. Even though in reality any love that can be defined in words is not love, for the sake of our current discussion let's overlook that fact for a while. There is considerable irony here because if we didn't ignore this fact, we would be forced to go to the place beyond the mind – the place where love was hiding all along. Let's see if there is a way of getting to the place beyond words, but through the use of words, by pretending to define unconditional love.

For many people, unconditional love is a strong affection felt for someone or something. To other people, it is some form of barter system in which one person has something to give in exchange for what can be gotten from the other person. For still others, it is a feeble way of disguising their fear of loneliness, isolation, and the terror of the Abyss of perhaps discovering they are unlovable.

At the deepest level, being alone may bring up guilt about one's unconscious separation from God/Wholeness. Being in a relationship may seem to satisfy that discomfort and seem to fill the Abyss of loneliness. Little do they realize that by courageously facing the Abyss of loneliness, they may find Who They Really Are, and set in motion the potential to find the ideal relationship, and much more.

Unconditional love means loving everyone, regardless of what they have done. Sure, it is easy to love Jesus and Mother Theresa, but loving unconditionally includes everyone regardless of what they have done.

Forgiving and loving someone unconditionally does not mean you condone their actions. It means recognizing the Divine dance we play as we show each other the distortions on our lenses.

According to the greatest minds, religions and spiritual teachings, we live in a non-local, non-dualistic world in which there is no separation. There is only one consciousness. There is no one separate from you to love you.

As the saying goes, we've been "looking for love in all the wrong places." We have been looking for love outside ourselves when True Love can only be found inside.

Love has nothing to do with another person since all there is - is one consciousness looking into a holographic Hall of Mirrors. **When we find love within ourselves, we will find love in the reflected images.** So, contrary to the popular song lyric, love is not a "second-hand emotion."

Once we find this love within ourselves, it will feel natural to love, because it will be an expression of Who We Really Are.

It doesn't matter whether the "other person" loves us back. To believe we need the love of another person is to believe we are less than Whole and sets ourselves up for suffering.

If they don't love us back, we need to love ourselves some more. True love is the realization that we are the source of love. It is up to us to love ourselves, regardless of what is reflected back to us. Eventually, those reflected images will have no choice but to reflect this love back to us.......
not that that matters.

If this seems to take a great deal of effort, something is wrong. Love that requires a lot of effort is not true Love. When it is a true expression of Who We Are, it is completely effortless and joyful.

Although being in one-way relationships may seem to hurt, the more we are willing to embrace our true loving nature beneath this hurt, the greater will be our capacity to love even more.

We need not go out of our way to get hurt in order to increase our capacity for love. We need not <u>do</u> anything other than <u>be willing</u> to take empowered action from a place of choice, and not from a place of craving or resistance.

Since all there is - is one consciousness looking into a holographic Hall of Mirrors, what I am seeing is inherently my reflection. Therefore, real love has nothing to do with another person.

Embarrassing Confessions

To be quite frank, taking responsibility for what I saw in my Hall of Mirrors was not a pretty picture. Realizing that the chaos, murders, and suffering in the world are a reflection of my distorted lens was quite overwhelming. The more closely I examined each Frankenstein Monster, the uglier it became. This process helped me see how each Monster was created. This exercise is not for everyone. It requires 100% honesty and responsibility for everything we see.

I realized I could not say with certainty that if I had the opportunity to have more money than I can imagine, have sex with virtually whomever and whenever I want, and have the world bowing at my feet, that I would not be a narcissist. I must admit that I would at least be tempted to do whatever it took to get whatever I wanted, especially if I had been raised in a family in which this was methodically encouraged with all kinds of brainwashing and rituals at a very early age.

Realizing I was not the only one (within the one consciousness) with those deeply hidden and repressed desires, I began to understand why the world is the way it is. I also found that the more emotional charge I had about specific characteristics of certain people, the more they represented the parts of my shadow side that required the most work.

I found that once I forgave, and once I felt unconditional love and laughed at my thoughts about them, I felt free from ever needing to play this seemingly endless karmic game. I was no longer the victim, and they were no longer the Victimizer, and vice versa, from lifetime to lifetime.

I also found that the more I worked on the qualities of people that triggered me, the less emotional charge I had toward them.

I realized that, although The Global Elite seems to be the most influential people in the world, only those who feel most insecure would go to the extent they do to cover up their insecurity.

The Global Elite are insecure because they do not know Who They Really Are. They are profoundly out of alignment with our interconnected reality. They do not realize that they are the source of the power they seek. They may never experience the bliss that comes from rediscovering this interconnectedness. What a pity that people who seem to have so much often have so little of what really matters. Hopefully they will read books like this before it is too late for them, too late for those they lead, and too late for the entire planet.

But even though The Global Elite doesn't know I even exist, I offer them unconditional love. Love is the language the blind can see, and the deaf can hear. It makes no difference whether they can see or hear me. In addition to helping clean distortions on my lens, loving them brings me the Deep Inner Peace that results from rediscovering our interconnectedness.

For many years, I allowed The Global Elite to cause me to live a life of Hell.... until I realized that if I believe that Heaven and Hell depend on other people and circumstances, I would continue to live in Hell.

It may be tempting to shut off the T.V. and not read the news. It would be peaceful to ignore the Illusory World and believe that everything is "love and light." But for me, it is important to use The Illusion constructively - to heal the distortions on my lens that are preventing me from aligning with the light and power of God. The Illusion still has important lessons for me. Living in denial of The Illusion can eventually lead to much more suffering, as resisting the "Illusory World" causes it to grow more frightening distortions.

Within The Illusion, I may seem like someone outside of you – someone who wrote this book to help you Awaken from the Illusory World. But because the world is composed of a Hall of Mirrors, I represent the part of your mind that is already Awake. And just as I live in your mind, so does everything else.

The Upside-Down Universe

We were conditioned to see others as separate from us in the same way we were conditioned to perceive the world as right side up, even though scientists have shown that images are focused on the retinas of our eyes upside down. If we were to start wearing prism glasses, at first we would perceive objects as being upside down, but after about two weeks, our perceptions would automatically conform to our conditioning, and once again, we would see things as right side up. **Conditioning overrides reality.**

It's the same as perceiving ourselves as a separate body. We are conditioned to perceive separation, even though in reality, this is "upside-down thinking." **We are conditioned to change our whole way of seeing our world to coincide with the consensus reality, whether or not this "reality" contradicts the true reality.**

If the consensus reality were that the world is flat, we would believe the world is flat. If the consensus is that we are a victim of the world, that is how we will create our reality. If the consensus reality is that we are a separate individual who doesn't deserve the loving and nurturing of others, that is the way we would perceive our world, regardless of how much this contradicts the truths we uncovered from quantum physicists and the core of religions.

We are each essentially one cell in this giant organism we call humanity. If we hate Hitler or any Victimizer in our life, we are expressing hatred toward ourselves. How can we feel lovable when we feel hatred toward a part of ourselves? This hatred toward ourselves is the reason we may feel unlovable. It is the driving force behind this car-ma. Car-ma is what drives many negative behaviors and what can drive people insane.

Many negative consequences result from feeling unlovable. Until the need to feel lovable is filled, we may never feel complete. Feeling unlovable is also a source of the cravings for sex, drugs, and most of our other cravings.

The reason we sometimes feel unlovable is because we don't recognize that there is no one else "out there" that is separate from us. We are the source of love. None of our reflections can reflect love unless we show them the love we would like reflected. When we find love within ourselves, we will find love in the reflected images.

If we were to see others through interconnected eyes, we would experience peace and nourishing neurotransmitters. This is the way we can approach the Hitlers in our life. We may not agree with their actions, but Who They Really Are is not their actions. Their Essence is the same Essence that is within you, me, and everyone else. If we resist that Essence, we cut ourselves off from the Totality of Who We Are.

Using my allegory, Hitler is a reflection of a massive distortion on our lens. If we judge that distortion, we are judging and condemning a vital part of us. If, however, we see him through interconnected eyes, we are realigning with our true nature that is necessary for our Wholeness. This part is required to make us Wholly Holy and powerful creators of our reality.

To help find our way out of our Illusory World and into the power that results from rediscovering our Wholeness, we must discern instead of judge, forgive instead of suffer, and offer unconditional love to the Hitlers in our life.

The Hitlers we most despise are our greatest teachers of unconditional love. Mother Theresa and Jesus uttered words that have changed relatively few. All the Hitlers in our lives provide us with powerful experiential lessons of what the greatest spiritual masters spoke – words that may have gone in one ear and out the other. Our Hitlers give us the opportunity to forgive and find pure unconditional love for them, to help us heal our shadow side. They are giving us the chance to experience "Forgive them Father for they know not what they do." They are giving us the opportunity to say, "Thy Will, not my will."

Only after we surrender entirely to "Thy Will," will we be able to take empowered action from The Zone. When we feel unconditional love for our Hitlers, we are much closer to healing our shadow side and feeling unconditional love for ourselves. Love helps dissolve our illusion of separation. It helps us laugh at our Illusion of Hell to enable us to live in The Zone.

"Humanity has unquestionably one really effective weapon—laughter...Against the assault of laughter, nothing can stand."
— Mark Twain

Chapter Thirteen
Entering The Zone at the Speed of Laughter

Let's face it. We live in a hedonistic, fast food culture in which change needs to happen in a New York minute, and where spending five minutes in meditation is considered overly self-indulgent. We want to go to the take-out window of our nearest ashram to get a supersized download of Buddha-nature-delight.

Well, I have good news for you. Our most overwhelming challenges are not only our greatest teachers; they are the catalysts for the quickest change. They drive us to the extreme right upper corner of our flow chart at the speed of laughter, which we will discuss in chapter 19.

Our most overwhelming challenges also do their best to force us down our emotional scale at the speed of tears. They are giving us the greatest opportunities to see the difference in results when we use "Power" (emotional levels 1 - 4) versus "Force" (levels 5 - 28).

Abraham Hicks[1] and David Hawkins[2] each have very helpful scales. The following scale is a way of combining their work in a novel way.

EMOTIONAL SCALE
Power
1. The Zone
2. Joy/Bliss/Freedom/Unconditional Love/Reverence/Peace/ Excitement/ Enthusiasm/ Empowerment/Happiness
3. Trust
4. Courage

Force

5. Positive Expectation
6. Optimism
7. Hopefulness
8. Contentment
9. Boredom
10. Pessimism
11. Irritation/Frustration
12. Overwhelmed
13. Doubt
14. Worry
15. Discouragement
16. Anger/Hate
17. Revenge
18. Rage
19. Jealousy
20. Insecurity/Guilt/Unworthiness
21. Fear/Depression/Powerlessness/Anxiety
22. Grief/Regret
23. Apathy/Despair
24. Guilt/Blame
25. Shame/Humiliation
26. Hopelessness and Helplessness
27. Surrender
28. The Great Abyss

Surrendered States

29. Death of conditioned thought (death of the ego)
30. Freedom from conditioned thought
31. The Zone

Many of us react to challenging people or situations by tending to gravitate to a particular level on this scale. This reaction may be in a Powerful way - levels 1–4, or in a Forceful approach - levels 5–28.

Most of us are very familiar with the use of force. It is often used as a means of protection, guarding an underlying sense of weakness. It is commonly used by default as a substitute for power or as a guard against weakness. We use force when we are essentially saying "my will, not Thy Will." The further down the emotional scale we are toward #28, the more mesmerized we are by the Illusory World, the more power we lose, and the more force we need to compensate for this loss. This is because the lower we go in the scale, the more we are forgetting to laugh, and the more out of alignment we are with God's Will.

Our culture seems to encourage us to use a forceful approach toward challenging people and situations. We are all familiar with the more obvious "forceful" approaches to challenges, such as pushy or manipulative confrontations and violence. Other "forceful" approaches are not so obvious - such as affirmations, visualizations, and reading or listening to spiritual talks in order to resist obstacles. People who use this more subtle forceful approach to "spirituality" rarely listen or watch the news for fear that would take them down the emotional scale toward the Great Abyss.

This "spiritual" forceful approach may be very successful in many situations. The problem is, this approach requires a great deal of effort if what we want is something that is out of alignment with "God's Will." If these spiritual approaches are used to resist "God's Will" they may not be successful in the long term, and that's a good thing in the bigger picture.

An alternative is to use the "powerful" approach. This approach is aligned with "God's Will" and can enable us to take a huge leap up the emotional scale - from the lowest emotions to those of Bliss/Freedom/ Unconditional Love/Reverence and Peace at the "speed of thought."

It is essential to keep in mind that Unconditional Love at Level 2 means loving everyone regardless of what they have done.

Although it may seem repulsive, this means unconditionally loving all the most appalling people in the world. This is a massive leap up the scale for many people. If you find this too challenging to do right now, please skip to the next section.

But if you feel empowered and courageous, and want to take a quick leap up the emotional guidance scale, going from the lowest emotional level to the highest at "the speed of thought," let's look at how you can redefine your challenges.

Redefine and Shine

When you are able to redefine people and situations in a way that enables you to feel the emotions closest to Level 1 on the scale, you will shine. You do this by experiencing true joy, gratitude and other Level 2 emotions toward challenging people for giving you the opportunity to clear another distortion on your lens. You will feel love toward them for taking on this challenging role as your teacher of unconditional love. You will feel a sense of freedom for no longer having the highly toxic neurotransmitters created by anger and judgments in your body.

All these ways of redefining challenging people and situations allow you to powerfully clear away more distortions on your lens and enables the Light of God to shine directly onto your Hall of Mirrors, allowing you to experience more Heaven in your life.

Another way to make this giant leap at "the speed of laughter" is by laughing at any thoughts that interfere with experiencing appreciation and gratitude toward our challenging Monsters using the many approaches in this book. The resulting Appreciation, Bliss, and Peace take us from the lower emotional levels to the Level 2 emotional level of Joy/Bliss and Freedom, at the speed of laughter.

Many spiritual teachers speak about the power of gratitude and love. These qualities are powerful because every time we feel gratitude or love we take a quick and giant leap up the emotional levels. These emotional leaps can bring about dramatic healing abilities in a virtual heartbeat.

One way to take this giant leap in our daily life is through communication. When someone does something that tickles us to have a negative emotion, we can use it in a positive way as follows:

Ho-Ho-Holy Communication

What follows is how I sometimes respond to people I know well who trigger me:

When you did/said _____ (describing the action or the statement as objectively as possible),

It triggered me to laugh at my thoughts about it. For this, I am very grateful.

I have a need to laugh at my thoughts.

In the future, you may want to laugh at your thoughts as well.

If I say these words without truthfully feeling and embodying them, the other person will see right through the scripted formula and will laugh **at me**.

The advantage of this form of communication is that it doesn't try to covertly manipulate the other person or give the other person any perceived power to influence my emotions in any way. That communication would imply that the other person has the power to change how we feel and that they need to feel guilty and change their behavior. The Ho-Ho-Holiest Communication demonstrates that the other person's behavior will only change in a way that meets my approval when I change myself. This is because we are all interconnected. The other person's behavior reflects what is going on within me at some deep level, regardless of how intensively I may resist this deeply repulsive fact.

Sometimes this Ho-Ho-Holy Communication involves the other person staying exactly the same, while I work much harder at laughing at my own thoughts about them. In this scenario, once I change my thoughts about them, I will see their behavior from an empowered place. I may then take empowered action from a place of choice.

Although this is a script, this communication is much more about the feeling expressed than about the spoken words. It is about internalizing the feeling in the deepest way and allowing the words to be passively spoken as an expression of the feeling.

It is not about communication through words, it is about allowing the gratitude for the laughter to express itself into words. I am expressing the feeling, not the words.

When I effectively use this approach, I often go from anger to joy at the speed of laughter.

The Joke Embedded in the Emotional Scale

By now you may have noticed the Joke/irony in this scale. There have been many emotional scales recorded throughout the years. This one is an expanded version based on some of the others. The irony of the scale can be seen in this expanded version. As we will see later, Jokes based on irony are typical of God's sense of humor.

The Joke is that whether we go to the top of the scale or to the bottom of the scale, we end up in exactly the same place - The Zone - in which there is the absence of conditioned thoughts. We find ourselves in a state of complete surrender to the Will of God and the infinite power it contains.

I had been working diligently for over 30 years to work my way up the scale, one step at a time in a diligent effort to one day make it to the top. I believed by ascending this scale that somehow, in some future lifetime, I would be an ascended master. I had overlooked the fact that whenever I would try to take the next step up, I was attached to that goal and was resisting my present conditions. This resistance to the present conditions caused more distortions on my lens. Those distortions became additional chains binding me to the Illusion of Hell.

If I let go of the attachment to taking the next step up the ladder and accepted the present moment completely, while still holding a preference for reaching the top of the scale, I would have the experience of Joy, Appreciation, Empowerment, Freedom or Love, but it would still be filtered by thought. It would be the Illusory World version of those high scoring emotions, rather than the version of those Blissful emotions I experienced during my Vipassana meditation, which was free of thought.

In retrospect, the path through the Abyss and death of the ego were the paths I had unknowingly taken when I experienced no thoughts. I experienced this virtual death of my thought-constructed identity during my Vipassana meditation and my near-death experience in the sweat lodge ceremony. Spiraling downward through pain and agony, through worry, discouragement, anger, and on through the great Abyss led to the Bliss beyond words relatively quickly.

Surrendering to what is, living in the present moment, and letting go of attachment to the outcome are all ways of entering The Zone at level # 31 instead of at level # 1. Because we have free will, the path to # 31 seems uncomfortable. But as Neale Donald Walsch once said, "Life begins at the edge of your comfort zone."

Although we might believe that our free will helps us reach the top of the emotional scale, it may be our biggest obstacle. Insisting on our will being done takes us out of alignment with God's Will. It, therefore, creates a huge distortion on our lens and delays our entering The Zone.

Reaching the top of the emotional scale is not just a fun exercise that allows us to feel good. It also raises our vibration, clears our lens, and allows our internal changes to be reflected in the world.

The path through the Abyss was the path Jesus tried to teach us when he said to God, "Thy will, not My will" when he was nailed to the cross and was resurrected. Although there are many teachers of how to ascend the emotional scale, Jesus taught how to navigate the descending route through forgiveness and surrender. Perhaps instead of calling him an ascended master, we may want to call him a descended master - a master at surrendering to descending the emotional scale. Perhaps that is the way to eventually ascend and resurrect ourselves.

We don't hear much about the most advanced spiritual masters doing visualizations and affirmations in an effort to ascend the emotional scale in a linear fashion. Nor do we hear accounts of Jesus having Post It Notes on His mirrors saying, "I am the Son of God."

Perhaps we can more rapidly become an ascended master and enter The Zone more quickly by first becoming a master of *descending* – like Jesus did. Perhaps one way to become an ascended master is by first becoming a descended one. Maybe instead of thinking of the emotional scale as linear, we can think of it as circular - as we can see in The Hero's Journey. It is by going down into the Abyss that we recover the treasures of life.

"Where you stumble, there lies your treasure."
— Joseph Campbell

Chapter Fourteen
The Hero's Journey

Just as we may think we've discovered a secret shortcut out of our Illusion of Hell to become an ascended master, we discover it's not that easy. Most of us need to also experience The Hero's Journey[1], as described by Joseph Campbell and others, beginning in 1871 with anthropologist **Edward Burnett Tylor's** observations.

This *Hero's Journey through the Abyss* and the death of conditioned thoughts is not only for people who think they are on a spiritual path. Most everyone will eventually need to take the descending journey into the Abyss that you can see below. The difference is how we make our ascension, and whether the Hero's Journey and the Abyss can be bypassed altogether. One question is how we can make this very challenging Journey as enjoyable as possible.

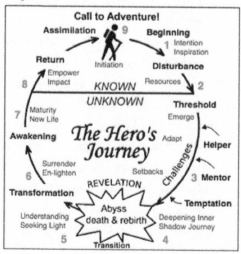

This is a description of the steps of the journey:

1. Beginning: The call to adventure. At first, the hero may refuse the call because of fears, duties or resistance. But if the hero refuses, she suffers, so she strives to do the right thing with intentions, aspirations, and inspiration for the journey ahead.

2. Resources: Acquiring spiritual teachings, magical crystals, unique gifts, objects, wisdom or any other "permission slips" that give the hero permission to deepen into the True Power that comes when the hero knows and embodies Who They Really Are.

3. Crossing the Threshold: The hero faces a maze of tests, challenges, and temptations that lead to finding some friends and enemies while harmonizing and adapting to setbacks along the way.

4. Deepening Inner Shadow Journey: Here, the hero confronts his disowned shadows, while preparing for the leap into the Abyss.

4 1/2.The Great Abyss: The Abyss may represent a dangerous physical test (e.g., illness, accident) or a spiritual crisis point (e.g., dark night of the soul). The hero goes through a death and rebirth process and is forever transformed.

5. Understanding: Insight, revelation or new knowledge acquired from this deepening through death and rebirth gives the hero a reward (e.g., secret, special power or insight). They refuse to go back to where they started, even though they may feel isolated and cut off from others and from themselves.

6. Surrendering: Facing challenges on the road back, the hero may feel threatened, but is rescued by listening to their newly acquired inner guidance. The challenge here is to develop the courage to surrender and be willing to let go of their attachment to worldly treasures, to listen to their inner guidance, and to surrender to a Higher Power.

7. Maturity: The hero learns to stop indulging in worldly distractions as she faces her new understanding of reality and her purpose in this reality. In this process, she starts a fresh new way of living with progressively less resistance. She becomes more purified and closer to a Higher Power. She lives more deeply in The Zone and is full of joy, spontaneity, and generosity.

8. Return home: Now the more self-actualized hero has gained mastery of more of the known and unknown worlds. They have wisdom to share in a way that impacts others and helps foster a new generation of heroes they mentor and empower.

9. Assimilation: Integration of all the experiences the hero has gained, as they settle into ordinary everyday life. The hero may still fall back into illusions and remain oblivious to their next deeper calling until they get shocked into entering a new cycle of adventure.

Steps 1 - 4 ½ of this journey are referred to as the *descension*. Steps 4 ½ - 9 are referred to as the *ascension*.

Some people on a spiritual path make their ascension by putting into practice what they have learned. They do their inner shadow work and learn to appreciate their shadows as their teachers. They learn to surrender and to accept life on life's terms. Life will always do an excellent job of letting us know whether the spiritual knowledge we've acquired is embodied and incorporated into our lives by the degree of joy or suffering we experience.

There are other people on the "everything is Love & Light" spiritual path who believe that affirmations and visualizations are the answer to life's challenges and the way to achieve The American Dream. This approach may indeed work for some people. Some try to achieve the American Dream as part of their efforts to resist falling into the Abyss.

Still others continue to resist the Abyss and keep suffering, without additional transformational tools. Some are so stuck in fight/flight/freeze mode, they don't even think about using their skills.

Life may continue giving them tools, but they insist on using tools they know are not working for them. They are so afraid of facing the Abyss that they get stuck suffering in their Illusion of Hell.

The more we refuse to face the Abyss with a peaceful heart, the more challenging our lessons may become. This is why the first three words of Lao Tzu's quote, "As soon as you have made a thought, laugh at it" are so important. It allows us to catch potential challenges before they become enormous challenges.

Embracing The Great Abyss

We can either come face-to-face with this Abyss by surrendering and embodying our spiritual teachings, through a near death experience, or through an actual death experience. Through one of these paths, we find that the Abyss we avoided like the plague was the greatest gift in helping us gain a deeper realization about the nature of reality and about Who We Really Are.

Resisting the Abyss is a root cause of suffering. This may continue until we learn that the Abyss is our friend. Again, this does not mean refraining from taking any action. It means taking empowered action from The Zone.

Our judgments about the Abyss cause our resistance and worsen our suffering. When experiencing the path down to the Abyss through the filters of thought, the journey can be quite frightening.

One powerful tool in this process is gratitude. When we can feel sincere gratitude for the transformational power of the Abyss, we immediately progress from the Abyss phase to the "Awakening" phase of our Journey. We go from the bottom of the emotional scale directly to the top.

A sign that we have been doing our work in laughing and surrendering is when we experience more synchronicities in our life. Many spiritual masters talk about their lives being synchronistic. Being on a "spiritual path" for many years, I wondered why I wasn't experiencing such synchronicities.

Then, one day I realized that since there is only one Consciousness, everything is happening synchronistically. The problem was, I wanted the world to respond on my terms with what I considered to be positive synchronicities, instead of on God's terms with God's synchronicities. This created a collision of opposing forces. One force was my will, desires, and resistances to what I didn't want. The other force was God's plan. When this conflict happens, we eventually, synchronistically, attract situations that cause us to face an Abyss that represents what we had been resisting.

The Abyss is presented to encourage our evolution. It is a synchronicity, just not one of our choosing. We therefore don't recognize it as a synchronicity. This grand Abyss is what many of us are experiencing in our world right now.

Once we surrender to the Abyss and to God's Will, we are in awe of all synchronicities. Then, life becomes an exciting adventure of synchronicity, discovery, and laughter at these discoveries!

Once we open to the grand picture, life is full of synchronicities.

If everyone were to laugh at the Most Powerful Joke, this could bring about the beginning of an appreciation of the Divinely planned Global synchronicity and would make our ascension from our global Abyss more powerful, transformational and enjoyable.

Instead, most of us come out of The Zone by resisting the Abyss, causing us to face a more challenging Hero's Journey - until we surrender.

My Hero's Journey

My Hero's Journey was a continual resistance of the Abyss by constantly running. I had been on a spiritual path for many years. After attending numerous workshops and reading many books about unconditional love, I foolishly believed I was a "master" of this topic.

Shortly after reading an excellent article on unconditional love, I saw a certain politician on T.V. My blood began to boil and felt as though my blood pressure was going through the roof. I felt enormous anger toward him and government corruption and deceit. I was so disgusted by the political system of the U.S. that I did my Dr. Skedaddle routine. I ran away as far as I could - to New Zealand.

At that point in my life, I had attained the American Dream. I had the nicest toys, a nice size bank account, the perfect loving relationship, and perfect medical practice, with excellent staff and lovely patients. To make that move meant surrendering essentially everything, not even knowing if I would be certified to practice medicine by their Medical Council. I decided to surrender my American Dream on a journey into facing my Abyss.

One day on a bike ride, it hit me like a ton of bricks. I was an "expert" on the topic of unconditional love, yet I felt overwhelming hatred toward this politician and the government.

At that moment, I had an epiphany: those people who made my blood boil were my greatest teachers of how to embody Unconditional Love. With that epiphany, I genuinely laughed at the Joke of it all. This was the revelation that inspired me to write this book.

While rewriting this book countless times over more than a decade, I was proud of the "final" version of the moment. One night, however, I received a not so subtle clue that I was not quite ready to expose myself by releasing my book. The night I completed that version of the book, I dreamt that I was walking naked in the middle of downtown Nelson, New Zealand, where I lived at the time. Passersby were staring at me as I meekly walked down the street in my birthday suit.

Despite this dream, I gave the manuscript to one of my friends to read. He verbally tore it apart and returned it to me after his cat had urinated on it.

Although I was initially humiliated by this, several months later I fully appreciated the cat's great wisdom. I had written meaningless words on paper only suitable for kitty litter.

The cat helped me realize I hadn't embodied the principles in the book and had remained in resistance to the Great Abyss. I hadn't surrendered to the possibility that after spending thousands of hours writing my most profound truths about a topic I felt very passionate about and that I believed was my soul's purpose to deliver, the only one who would enjoy my book would be a cat with a full bladder.

I decided that if I wanted to embody the principles in this book, I needed to leave New Zealand. This meant leaving a perfect relationship and a perfect job in a utopia to face a greater Abyss by returning to the U.S. This would force me to live in a state of inner peace right in the middle of a politically corrupt country and in the crosshairs of possible nuclear bombs. As crazy as that may sound, it was one of the best things I've done in my life.

If I had stayed in New Zealand and ignored everything I describe in this book, my continuing refusal to laugh at my Frankenstein Monsters would have been reflected back to me by readers refusing to laugh at their Monsters. They would have laughed at me instead. I realized that the only way for readers to laugh their way out of the Hall of Mirrors was for me to set the example and return to the U.S.

The process of facing my pain by learning its lessons during Vipassana is the same pattern I used when intentionally facing my fear of returning to the U.S.

I was forced to either suffer from my negative thoughts or surrender to the Abyss. I chose neither. Instead, I listened to Lao Tzu and decided to bypass the Hero's Journey. Instead, I chose laughter, which helped me to emerge transformed by my Abyss.

Most people face their Abyss by default. It may seem absurd to face our Abyss out of choice. But when there appear to be juicy lessons to learn by using this process, I sometimes find it helpful to use my scariest Frankenstein Monsters as my greatest transformational teachers.

I had done affirmations, visualizations, and mantras most of my life. I used countless "powerful" crystals, drums and magical fairy dust as "*permission slips.*" I subconsciously believed those permission slips would give me permission to deepen into my True Power. I failed to realize that this Power only comes when we know and embody Who We Really Are by facing our Abyss.

Mankind is on the precipice of a challenging Abyss, one that involves confronting The Inconvenient Joke. Our seemingly crazy world, full of horrific acts of terror, is providing us with a golden opportunity to do our Hero's Journey through this Abyss to be a descendant master. Our success in navigating this Abyss depends on how much we incorporate all that we have learned as we face our blockages to true Global abundance of mind, body, and spirit - in harmony with our planet. This Abyss may create the appearance of the loss of many of our possessions, whether by natural disasters or other circumstances, until one day we wake up and realize that our obsession with those possessions was possessing us.

As we surrender to the transformational nature of the Abyss and discover Who We Really Are beyond the Illusory World, we may find miracles and a Bliss beyond our wildest imagination. One way of joyfully facing the Abyss is by bypassing The Hero's Journey.

Bypassing The Hero's Journey

I have good news for you! Now that we know the rules, we are in a better position to break them.

The good news is: we need not spiral through the dark night of the soul nor through the Abyss. We need not be nailed to a cross, have a near-death experience, nor struggle to ascend the emotional scale. As I realized in my Hero's Journey, we can completely bypass the traditional Hero's Journey. All we need to do is laugh!

You read that right. Many people believe that following a spiritual path is difficult. They think it involves suffering and living in poverty. They believe that because "it is easier for a camel to go through the eye of a needle than for a rich person to enter the Kingdom of God," it is best to be poor. All this spiritual martyrism is only as valid as we make it with our beliefs.

The way to bypass the Abyss, the dark night of the soul, and this spiritual martyrism, is through laughter. Many spiritual teachings say that thoughts create things. For this reason, laughter, which brings us to the dimension beyond thoughts, would make it easy to pass through the eye of a needle because, without thoughts, nothing is preventing such passage. There is no separate needle's eye to pass through and no separate "I" that needs to pass through it. All there is, is the Kingdom of Heaven, in which everything is one unified soup of energy.

A similar situation would take place in The Hero's Journey. By laughing at our thoughts and at the Joke, we bypass conditioned thought. Without such thoughts, there is no resistance to reality, no belief in the need for magic crystals, no challenges or temptations, no disowned shadows, no perceived danger of facing the Abyss, no thoughts that would create any suffering on the way back, no cravings to be self-indulgent, and no shocks to enter new adventures. None of the stages of the Hero's Journey would exist.

By laughing at our thoughts, we may continue to cycle through our Hero's Journey. But instead of the Journey forcing this struggle, we remain peaceful and joyful, and quite amused by the process.

The trick is to do precisely as Lao Tzu said: "**As soon as** you have made a thought, laugh at it." Again, the first three words of this are key. The longer we wait before laughing at a thought, the further down the Hero's Path we go, and the more difficult it is to let go of our attachment to our journey and to the Illusion of Hell.

Beliefs that Interfere with This Laughter

1. We need someone or something to protect us from the evil people and situations of this cruel world.

Yes, there seem to be many evil people in the world who appear to be out to get us. But those evil people are the result of distortions we create in our continual battle to be safe. We are essentially saying to the world, "my will, not Thy Will," even though we know this is diametrically opposite from Jesus' teaching. It is amusing how many people who believe they are following Jesus' teachings have ignored one of His main teachings - one that he sacrificed his life to teach. It is fine to take action in response to some people and situations that we have not yet realized are our collective projections, as long as those actions are empowered and inspired by living in The Zone. Taking such empowered action is a natural byproduct of laughing at our fearful thoughts.

2. We need to do affirmations and visualizations.

It's okay to do affirmations and visualizations, but some people use them as a defense against facing the Abyss, again using the "my will, not Thy Will" approach. Although this approach may work for a while in coercing the Universe to manifest our demands, it may not be very effective in the long run because the distortions it creates on our lens will eventually need to be cleaned. Some of the imbalances we are witnessing in our world right now are consequences of the spiritual consumerism version of "my will, not Thy Will," and using affirmations and visualizations to get more stuff.

3. My family, my community, my church, my insurance, the police, the military will protect me.

Protect you from whom? There is only one consciousness, of which you are a part. This one consciousness is reflected back to you in your Hall of Mirrors. The more protection you crave, the more need for protection you may require.

Of course, if we laugh at our thoughts as a spiritual way of escaping the Abyss, then instead of escaping, our laughter causes us to be more imprisoned by our Illusory World - and the Joke's on us.

"Doctor, I have an earache.
"Here, eat this root."
"That root is heathen, say this prayer."
"That prayer is superstition, drink this potion."
"That potion is snake oil, swallow this antibiotic."
"Oops, bugs mutated. Here, eat this root!"
— A Short History of Medicine

Chapter Fifteen
Is Laughter the Best Medicine?

Norman Cousins was a long-time editor of the Saturday Review. He was a global peacemaker and received hundreds of awards, including the UN Peace Medal and nearly 50 honorary doctoral degrees.

In 1964, following a very stressful trip to Russia, he was diagnosed with Ankylosing Spondylitis. This left him in severe pain. He was told by his doctor that his health would never improve—that he would be bedridden and either in pain or so drugged that he wouldn't know what was going on around him, and that he would die within a few months.

Cousins noted that this disease began after a stressful trip to Russia. He disagreed with his doctor and believed that, if the harmful stresses of his trip had contributed to his illness, positive emotions and laughter could improve his condition.

With his doctors' consent, Cousins checked himself out of the hospital and into a hotel across the street. He obtained every Marx Brothers, Three Stooges, and other comedy tapes that he could lay his hands on and watched them continuously. He claimed that 10 minutes of belly laughter gave him two hours of pain-free sleep when nothing else – not even very high dose analgesics – could help him.

In a transcribed radio broadcast of August 1983 entitled, "Norman Cousins Talks on Positive Emotions and Health," Cousins described his research showing that the body produces its own Morphine -Enkephalins, and Endorphins. The brain also produces gamma globulin, which plays a role in strengthening the immune system. Also, the brain produces a substance known as interferon, which is an anti-viral agent and fights infections. Some medical researchers believe interferon also has a role in combating cancer.

Cousins found that laughing made his pain go away without the debilitating drugs. After some weeks of taking his own "cure," his condition steadily improved, and he slowly regained the use of his limbs. Within six months, he was back on his feet. Within two years, he was able to return to his full-time job at the Saturday Review. All he needed to do was sit back, relax, and allow the work to be done by "Doctors Moe, Larry, and Curly." It seems a bit ironic that a cure that couldn't be achieved by the best of modern medicine was achieved by three stooges.

Many believe his self-treatment is living proof that "laughter is the best medicine." Despite his demonstration, I'm not holding my breath for the day comedy is taught in medical schools. Although, maybe this book will help open that door.

Cousins' story baffled the scientific community because they were more focused on the blood pressure, pulse, and respirations as his vital signs. While these signs are vitally important, there is another vital sign often overlooked, namely a patient's ability to sees how their psycho-emotional state may have influenced their disease. The patient's ability to work together with their doctor (and their version of the Three Stooges) to change their underlying emotional state is often as important as the vital physical signs in indicating a prognosis.

Norman Cousins' story demonstrates the power of laughter for improving one's health. Watching comedy movies is very helpful in improving health, because laughter changes our biochemistry, as has been scientifically verified. But laughing at our thoughts and at the Powerful Joke can not only change our biochemistry, it can also help release the underlying thoughts that created toxic biochemistry. In so doing, it can help eliminate any psycho-emotional factors that may have contributed to the condition.

The ability for Norman Cousins and many others to heal from laughter is due to the mind/body connection. Norman realized that the stress from his trip to Russia was responsible for his Ankylosing Spondylitis. He recognized the mind/body connection and healed himself.

The Psychology of Disease

There is compelling medical research to suggest that many diseases, including cancer, may be influenced by psychological factors like stress, depression, hopelessness, and pessimism. There is a whole field of medicine, called psychoneuroimmunology, which studies the interaction between our psychological processes and the nervous and immune systems. Psychoneuroimmunology (PNI), also referred to as Psychoendoneuroimmunology (PENI), is the study of how the brain, nervous system, endocrine system, and the immune system all impact each other. It is now widely accepted in medical circles that chronic, persistent stress triggers many illnesses[1].

The specialty began as Psychoneuroimmunology (PNI). The letters "endo" were later added because the endocrine system was also found to play an important role, so it is sometimes called Psychoneuroendocrinology (PNEI). In a few years, I predict they will discover how all the bodily systems interact, and will add cardiology, gastroenterology, rheumatology, dermatology, orthopedics, gynecology, urology and hematology to the field, so the specialty will be called Psychoneuroendocardiogastrorheumatodermoorthogynourohematoimmunology. When that happens, it will be easier to forgive and love than to pronounce the doctor's specialty.

According to PENI, as we change our thoughts, we change our brain and thus our biology. Because of the relationship between our thoughts and our biology, researchers have found that different diseases are associated with different personality types.

There seems to be an "auto-immune disease personality." A French study compared 40 women who presented with auto-immune diseases, including systemic lupus erythematosus, scleroderma, polymyositis,

Sjögren's syndrome, vasculitis and mixed connective tissue diseases consisting of combined features of scleroderma, myositis, systemic lupus erythematosus, and rheumatoid arthritis, with a control group of 41 women without the auto-immune disease. The study showed that all 40 patients who had auto-immune diseases differed from the control group by their unobtrusiveness, self-deprecation, hyper-conformability and excessive kindness. There was a tendency toward contradiction and intolerance in patients with Sjögren's syndrome and a lack of aggressiveness combined with a feeling of inferiority in patients with vasculitis. The study confirmed that patients with auto-immune diseases are psychologically fragile and suggested that a psychological intervention should be examined[2].

The study also suggested that immune dysfunction may not be limited to these diseases. Research suggests that negative emotions stimulate proinflammatory cytokines that can contribute to a host of conditions associated with "normal" aging, including arthritis, cardiovascular disease, cancers, type 2 diabetes, functional decline, and frailty[3].

Multiple Sclerosis, Parkinson's and Alzheimer's may also have an auto-immune basis[4, 5, 6]. These, like the other auto-immune diseases, may be helped with psychological interventions.

There is also a Type A personality type described as ambitious, rigidly organized, impatient, highly status-conscious – one who takes on more than they can handle, is anxious, and concerned with time management. They are often high-achieving "workaholics" who push themselves with deadlines and can't bear delays. Type A personality types are more likely to have hypertension, heart attacks, and strokes.

A "Type C Personality" is described as the "Cancer Personality." They are often depressed, angry and afraid to express their emotions. Type C's are the polar opposite of Type A's. Type C's are un-emotional, non-assertive, and appease others to the point of self-effacement and self-sacrifice. Type C's may have an increased risk of cancer[7].

Some oncologists are uncomfortable with discussing the idea of a cancer personality because they believe patients will think they brought the disease on themselves. They say the research is inconclusive in any case.

But if someone really wants to heal, there is no room for blaming oneself or anyone else. I feel great compassion for anyone with cancer. The idea of a cancer personality and entertaining the possibility that you caused this life-threatening illness can be extremely frightening. If you think the possibility that you brought on the cancer yourself is too painful to accept, then please ignore everything I am about to say. If you find this line of exploration unpleasant, I am sorry for bringing it up.

The Psychology of Health

But if you believe your mental and emotional state might have that much power to cause the cancer, you must also have that much power to let it go!

Many studies in mainstream journals acknowledge this link between our emotions and cancer. According to an article in the European Journal of Cancer, there is substantial evidence linking abnormalities in immune function with psychological stress. The research concluded that psychological and behavioral factors may influence the incidence or progression of cancer. The study found that the possibility that psychological interventions may improve immune function and survival among cancer patients clearly merits further investigation[8].

In his book, *Prescriptions For Living*, Dr. Bernie Siegel found that long-term cancer survivors were those who paid attention to their feelings, expressed their emotions and became more spiritual. I highly recommend this and his other book, *Love, Medicine, and Miracles*, for people with intractable diseases[9].

A study of women with metastatic breast cancer was published in the prestigious medical journal, Lancet. It found that stress reduction and social support proved more beneficial for improving quality of life and symptom control than for those who received only medical treatment. More importantly, it also resulted in them living longer[10]!

Bringing this back to my allegory, cancer and other diseases are frightening Frankenstein Monsters that seem as though they are out to get us. It can be very distressing to admit how those frightening reflections arose, but once we do, we regain control of our condition.

While some oncologists say there is inconclusive research on the role of psychological interventions on cancer survival, the fact is, there is CONCLUSIVE, "gold-level" evidence from three randomized control studies involving a total of 271 patients, showing that arthroscopic debridement for knee arthritis is NOT helpful, yet it is extensively being done[11].

If procedures are being done that are proven to not be helpful for non-life-threatening conditions, do we want to wait for more people to die before considering virtually risk-free psychological interventions for life-threatening conditions when these psychological interventions have been proven to be more beneficial in improving quality of life and in extending life span than some medical interventions?

Some people believe that psychological interventions are useless for medical conditions because many diseases are determined by our DNA over which we have no control.

This is certainly what we have been taught to believe. We are told by "those who know" that humans are nothing more than the calculated, deterministic expression of our genes; helpless robots whose biology, emotions and health are determined by our DNA over which we have no control.

The Inconvenient Dogma of Biology

The central dogma of Biology is also called the Holy Grail of Medicine. It states that information in our cells flows from DNA to RNA to proteins. This Holy Grail implies that we are pitiful victims of our DNA and are therefore dependent on pharmaceuticals for our health. We are born with these latent diseases and are unable to change their inevitability.

This was a very inconvenient dogma for humans, but a very convenient dogma for the pharmaceutical companies. This theory is still being taught in medical schools and universities all over the world.

For those who still believe in this Holy Grail, I have two questions:

1. How is it possible for bacteria grown in different Petri dishes with different culture media to change their characteristics if the bacteria in each dish has fixed genetic material?

2. When studying identical twins, how is it possible for one twin to have a disease while the other twin is entirely normal as determined by many studies, including a study out of The University of Utah[12]?

The only way for either of these questions to be answered is to admit that our gene expression can be modified. As Dr. Bruce Lipton points out, our genes are like a blueprint. A builder can follow the blueprint precisely as it is in the plans or decide to rip it up and follow a completely different blueprint.

Because I went through medical school never questioning what I was taught, I never bothered, until recently, to look up the word "dogma." I found dogma defined as "A belief taught by a religious organization and accepted by the members of a group without being questioned or doubted."

In his autobiography, *What Mad Pursuit*, Francis Crick wrote about his choice of the word dogma. "I used the word the way I myself thought about it, not as most of the world does, and simply applied it to a grand hypothesis that, however plausible, had little direct experimental support."

Cellular biologist Dr. Bruce Lipton, Ph.D. is one of the leading authorities on how emotions can regulate genetic expression. He has written excellent books including "*The Biology of Belief*," and "*Spontaneous Evolution*." Dr. Lipton and many others have shown that the central dogma of DNA inevitability is false. Genes alone do not determine human outcomes, nor do environmental circumstances. Our *responses* to our DNA and our environment are what actually determine the expression of our genes.

I was astounded to realize this Holy Grail of medicine on which we base much of our dependency on medications has little direct experimental support. In contrast, the importance of using laughter as medicine is proven with studies, though not widely accepted. The main difference in accepting the Central Dogma and in accepting the power of laughter is that laughter is a potentially healing dogma as it may help modify our DNA expression with no negative side-effects. Modifying our DNA expression means instead of believing that we are a victim of our genes, we can have designer genes.

One way to explain how it is possible that our genes alone don't determine our propensity for disease is through an understanding of epigenetics. Epigenetics is the study of how our genes are influenced by external or environmental factors that switch genes on and off. This means that we are not controlled by our genes. Whether genes are turned on or off is primarily determined by our thoughts, beliefs, attitudes, perceptions and environmental exposures.

As you may know, stress and negative emotions result in a reduction in serotonin and dopamine levels in the brain. They also raise cortisol, insulin, and bad cholesterol levels, leading to depression, endocrine and immune system dysfunction, resulting in a variety of diseases.

As we know from PNI, our immune and endocrine systems are always eavesdropping on our emotional wellbeing. These systems are essentially behaving like the CIA. They are essentially conducting wiretaps to make sure no negative emotions are behaving like evil terrorists. The problem is that our weapons of mass distraction, like alcohol, drugs or un-needed food, together with anxiety, anger, and fear producing news reports allow our emotional terrorists to remain well disguised and undetectable, except in the illnesses they quietly cause. Allowing negative emotions to continue to go undetected gives these emotional terrorists the ability to plant bombs in strategic places, such as in the heart. When these bombs are ignited - often by stress - disease erupts.

Another avenue for negative emotions to carry out terrorist acts is when these emotions hijack our personality. This could result in an auto-immune personality or an A or C type personality. Because these personality types are considered normal and the resulting emotions are often silenced by alcohol, drugs or food, the terrorists often remain concealed.

Believing that we are victims of our genes, we may think there is nothing we can do for our health other than relying on pharmaceutical companies for our health.

Once we dare to laugh at our thoughts responsible for these different personality types which in turn are responsible for these diseases, we realize that we are no longer a victim of our genes, but the master of them.

Now that the "Central Dogma of Biology" has been officially disproven, is it possible that the dogma that says we are a victim of our Hall of Mirrors is the next dogma to be officially disproven? I am not suggesting a total abandonment of our current dogma, as this may seem extremely challenging. I am merely suggesting that one helpful way to uncover hidden saboteurs of health is to conduct our own research and to QUESTION EVERYTHING you've been told, including what I say in this book.

Questioning everything also includes questioning the permanence of one's personality type, opening the door to new ways of perceiving and responding to your world.

Treating Root Causes of Disease for the Best Results

Studies show there can be continuing personality changes even through late adulthood[13]. The cancer personality trait can be changed. For someone with cancer, in addition to following your doctor's recommendations regarding chemotherapy and radiation, it is important to thoroughly research all other available treatments and consider additional options, including following an anti-cancer diet. In addition to following a special diet of the food you ingest, it is essential to follow a special diet of the thoughts and beliefs you ingest, remembering that….. "in–jesting" is the best way to take in everything.

There are also studies showing that cancer survival may improve with hypnotherapy[14, 15, 16].

A disease is a scary Frankenstein Monster which deserves medical attention as well as Powerful Laughter about any root emotional causes. It can often take intensive work to finally find that Laughter, but when we do, it can be extremely transformational. Since the negative emotions and resulting behaviors are often passed on for many generations, our Laughter can be transformational for future generations.

From a PNI perspective, forgiving and unconditionally loving everyone who challenges us can significantly help our immune system function more effectively to optimize its response to cancers and other diseases. From an epigenetic perspective, since cancer is a function of how our genes are expressed, having positive thoughts, beliefs, attitudes, and perceptions can improve our genetic expression.

In addition to all the challenging people in our lives, the most important person to forgive and unconditionally love is ourselves. Once we have healthy thoughts and are in alignment with the Light of God, the reflections in our Hall of Mirrors will reflect a healthy body back to us.

There is a hierarchy in treating medical conditions. When we treat a medical condition with a modality such as surgery, at best we are curing the most superficial level of the condition. When we treat a medical condition with medications, at best we are curing both the intermediate level and superficial level. When we treat a medical condition with a modality such as hypnosis, at best we are curing the superficial, intermediate and deep levels. When we treat a medical condition with *LaughGnosis*, a process that combines laughter at the Powerful Joke with hypnosis in order to know the God Healer within us, at best, we may be able to cure our superficial, intermediate, deep and deepest levels on a longer-term basis, and can pass this healing power on to future generations. (*LaughGnosis* will be further described in Chapter 23.) To some, helping to cure disease by changing our personality, along with medications prescribed by your doctor if and as needed, may be considered a miracle. Most of us believe we are incapable of miracles, but is that really true?

"There are only two ways to live your life. One is as though nothing is a miracle. The other is as though everything is a miracle."
— Albert Einstein

Chapter Sixteen
Miracles

Have you ever wondered how Jesus performed miracles? Have you ever wanted to perform miracles like Jesus? Have you ever thought that the only hope for humanity is a miracle? Well, by the end of this chapter you will have a better idea of how Jesus may have performed miracles and how it may be possible to experience miracles even greater than those told in the stories of Jesus.

As we saw in chapter 6, according to *A Course in Miracles*, a miracle is a correction in perception. Through that change of thought, miracles can happen. A miracle "does not create nor change anything at all." Since the world is a reflection of our thoughts and perceptions, nothing needs changing other than our perception and thoughts. According to my allegory of the mirrors, for God's light to shine miracles onto our Hall of Mirrors, our lens needs to be as clean as possible.

If we try to create miracles, we may fail. When the act of trying to create a miracle puts us out of alignment with what is happening, this only creates more distortions on our lens. Therefore, instead of trying to *create* miracles, we can *experience* God's miracles by using five powerful alchemical tools. These alchemical tools are:

1. Forgiveness
2. Unconditional love
3. Knowing the true nature of reality
4. Knowing the truth of Who We Really Are
5. Laughter

As we have seen, **forgiveness** and **unconditional love** are two of the best lens cleaners.

If we merely follow a formula for experiencing miracles and don't understand its underlying rationale, it is less likely to work, and we are not likely to follow through. But once we understand and use my allegory as a map of our non-local reality and as a way to make sense of our chaotic world, we are more likely to use it effectively. As we do, we will see our challenges in a positive framework. The more we can welcome our challenges, the more distortions on our lens we will dissolve and the more miracles we will experience.

Another alchemical tool for experiencing miracles is **knowing Who We Are**. Knowing who are we goes beyond who we think we are. It goes beyond any identification of ourselves as our occupation, beliefs, and our body.

"Know Thyself," was the maxim at the Temple of Delphi. At the threshold of the Temple, a Greek maxim was engraved in the stone. It stated: *Homo Nosce te Ipsum,* which means "Man know thyself and thou shalt know the Universe and the Gods."

Knowledge of oneself is the only real knowledge. Only when we understand ourselves can we truly understand another. This is why the Oracle of Delphi proclaimed to "know thyself," for within each of you, all is contained.

Mohammed also said, "He who knows his own self, knows God" and Lao Tzu said, "Knowing others is wisdom; knowing yourself is Enlightenment."

Knowing Who We Are gives us the ability to live beyond this Illusory World we call reality. But until we can laugh at The Illusion, all these lovely words can merely be another form of mind game. Once we laugh at how seriously we are playing a locality game of believing in the possibility of separation in a non-local and perfectly united Universe, the game of locality is over. But knowing Who We Are within the non-local world in which everything is interconnected and laughing at how seriously we respond to our reflections can be challenging. We are highly conditioned to believe that everyone and everything is separate. When we look at the Hall of Mirrors, we realize that although there is only one of us looking into the mirrors, over seven billion reflections are looking back. Which one of them is us?

When we think about it, it is a bit like the movie "Sybil" about a woman who had 16 different personalities.

The way we act in our world is similar in some ways to how Sybil acted in her world. We seem to live in a dysfunctional Sybilization in which Sybil could serve as our role model.

Sybil was diagnosed with a multiple personality disorder; she had only 16 different personalities and was considered insane. The civilization of humanity has seven billion personalities, with 384,000 new personalities born each day, yet we are considered sane.

Miracles are happening all around us that are often disguised and dismissed merely because they seem haphazard. As you will see in the next section, once we are consciously able to master these principles, we may be able to experience miracles.

Miracles in Disguise

As previously stated, a miracle is an event that provokes wonder, because it is contrary to our expectations and appears to be unexplainable.

Whether or not something is a wonderful event depends more on the perceiver than what is being perceived. For most people, waking up to a sunrise on a tropical beach in the Cayman Islands might be wonderful; a pile of feces might be disgusting. But in the eyes of someone seeing their last sunrise before being executed, that sunrise would be horrifying, while in the eyes of a person with chronic constipation, there can be no better miracle than a wondrous bowel movement.

Miracles are happening all around us, but we sometimes don't notice or appreciate them.

These miracles can best be seen in people with multiple personality disorders, more officially known as "dissociative identity disorders."

Different personality states of people with "dissociative identity disorders" display differences in dominant handedness in response to the same medication, allergic sensitivities, and blood flow to the brain, as well as differences in visual acuity, eye curvature, pupil size, and eye pressure[1].

Dr. Francine Rowland, a Yale psychiatrist who specializes in treating people with dissociative identity disorders, tells about a person who was stung by a wasp. His eye was swollen shut and he was in severe pain. Rowland hypnotized the patient into letting an anesthetic personality with insensitivity to pain take control of his body, and the eye returned to normal[2].

Often one or several of a multiples' personalities are children. If an adult personality is given a drug like Valium and then a child's personality takes over, the adult dosage may be too much for the child and result in an overdose. Frequently personalities will have different handwriting, artistic abilities or even knowledge of foreign languages. There can also be an abrupt appearance and disappearance of rashes, welts, scars and other tissue wounds or switches in handwriting and handedness or epilepsy, allergies and color blindness that strike only when a given personality is in control of the body[3].

Although many people still believe that depression is due to a serotonin deficiency, in 1983 the National Institute of Mental Health (NIMH) concluded that "There is no evidence that there is anything wrong in the serotonergic system of depressed patients."

I believe that depression may not be caused by a serotonin deficiency, but by a laughter deficiency. Instead of taking medications to correct a normally functioning serotonin system, all that may be necessary is to laugh at the Inconvenient Joke and trigger a healthier and happier personality.

One person with a dissociative identity disorder was admitted to a hospital for diabetes and baffled her doctors by showing no symptoms when one of her non-diabetic personalities was in control[4].

There are also accounts of epilepsy coming and going with changes in personality[5].

It's interesting to examine these cases because they make it perfectly clear that seemingly "permanent" conditions and diseases of the body are being cured through the mind alone, in a matter of minutes.

Diabetes, poor eyesight, color blindness, knowledge of foreign languages, epilepsy, allergies, eye curvature, response to medications, scars, burn marks, handedness, etc. all seem to be fixed conditions. But these multiple personality cases indicate it is the mind that is the cause of these conditions. They can change with a shift in thought that triggers a different personality. Nothing was done to them at the physical level.

We are conditioned to believe that there is a genetic basis to color blindness, diabetes, and epilepsy, and that they could not change with a change in personality. This belief, however, may be a factor causing medical conditions to be more difficult to treat, considering what we know of Epigenetics.

Modifying Genetic Diseases

Many people believe that since genetics is the cause of their disease, they have no control over it and need to stay on medication for the remainder of their lives. Through our understanding of epigenetics, psychoneuroimmunology, personality types, and dissociative identity disorders, we know this is not necessarily the case.

Shifts from a disease state to a healed, normal state and vice-versa occur most often in people with dissociative identity disorders, because they are outside the rules of genetics, and don't consider for a moment the possibility that such changes are not possible. They don't say, hold on a moment, I need to check my family genetics before letting go of my tumor. They just let them go.

The problem is that many "normal and intelligent" adults are too intelligent to allow miracles to happen, because of their highly conditioned, limiting beliefs. They are conditioned to believe that if they have bad vision, epilepsy, or a tumor, they will have this condition forever. They do not consider that it may be possible to change these "permanent" conditions with a change in mood, thought or belief. Once limiting beliefs are dissolved, miracles are much more likely.

The ability of people with dissociative identity disorders to go between normal and diseased states very quickly demonstrates the human potential, but from this glimpse into the reality behind our beliefs, we must learn how to gain conscious control.

Many of the changes result from shifting into a personality that is more adapted to a particular situation. For instance, the personality with the tumor may be more adapted to the personality that no longer wishes to live while the personality that is tumor free sees their tumor as their teacher, learns its lessons and has a renewed outlook on life. If they don't learn their lessons from the tumor in this life, they may have similar challenges in their next life - until they clear the distortion on their lens that was causing the tumor.

The diseases that we now believe are physical, although they may sometimes require medications or surgery, can sometimes be effectively treated at the level of the mind. When diseases are treated at the level of the mind, not only can the disease improve, but associated symptoms can also often improve.

These psychological changes can be accomplished through processes like *LaughGnosis*, in which the practitioner is first able to laugh away their own blockages to their authentic laughter and laugh themselves to health - and then help the patient to do the same. This process can help the patient associate into a healthy personality, having learned what they needed to learn from the diseased personality. A health practitioner who can use these principles can often allow miracles to happen!

This will be discussed in more length in our discussion about using the *Mitote* for miracles in chapter 20. But suffice it to say for now that there is a fine line between what is considered a manifestation of a dissociative identity disorder and a miracle. The difference is in the ability to control the changes by regaining awareness of our holographic Hall of Mirrors.

The first step in regaining this awareness and experiencing miracles is Knowing Ourselves. Since we are created in God's image, to know ourselves is to know God. And since God can create miracles, by knowing Who We Are, we will be better able to see more miracles all around us.

One example of this was during the ten-day meditation program in which I took 100% responsibility for my pain. In this process, I corrected my perception until I saw pain as my teacher who helped me to experience my pain from a very Blissful perspective. This correction in perception is the definition of a miracle according to the book, *A Course in Miracles.* It allowed me to experience the miraculous transformation of my excruciating pain to Bliss beyond imagination – quite an epiphany for this pain relief doctor!

Irony Deficiency/God's Humor 101

In addition to correcting our perception by seeing our Frankenstein Monsters as our teachers, we can correct our perception by seeing God's ironic Jokes in our everyday life.

If Voltaire is right and God is "a comedian playing to an audience too afraid to laugh," irony and paradox seem to be His comedy style.

The reason for the appearance of ironies and paradoxes is because we live in a world in which cause and effect are completely reversed. We believe the world is the cause of our suffering when the distortions in our lens are the cause of what we see in our world.

We live in a world that appears upside down on our retina, although we perceive it right side up. We have a dualistic perspective of a non-dualistic/non-local world.

Our perception is diametrically contradictory to reality. Thus, it seems only logical to see the resulting ironies, paradoxes and God's comedy show wherever we go. The reality we imagine is very different from true reality. Ironies and paradoxes bring to our attention the incongruity between true reality and the reality we imagine in a way that is so completely reversed that it is quite funny.

Our world is full of ironies. Even the Hero's Journey is a big irony. We resist the great Abyss like the plague, yet it is the most significant step in our transformation.

Many people suffer because they don't see the ironies all around them. They suffer from *irony deficiency*. Unfortunately, this is not something treatable by one doctor..........it requires treatment by a paradox.

Laughing at ironies and paradoxes is a way of busting ourselves for playing along and allowing ourselves to be fooled by the "Illusory World," in a very powerful yet non-judgmental way that bypasses the logical mind.

Here are some examples of ironies and paradoxes that seem typical of God's sense of humor:

- Fear of death prevents us from being fully alive.
- Our worst enemy is often our greatest teacher.
- Enjoying the journey is the goal.
- "Nothing" contains everything.
- "Nothing" lasts forever.
- "Nothing" is sacred.
- "Nothing" is a miracle.
- "Nothing" is better than sex.
- The Great Abyss - our worst nightmare - is the gateway to freedom.
- Pain can result in Bliss beyond words.
- The best way to Awaken is to catch ourselves asleep.
- The answer is to ask the right questions.
- One way to find enlightenment is to stop searching.
- Take The Joke seriously.
- Crazy people who are happy are put into funny farms by neurotic and depressed people who are considered to be "sane."
- Calling something a problem is part of the problem.
- The problem (i.e., the Abyss we fear) is the solution.

The way the problem is the solution is a result of a labeling issue. Labeling something as a problem and something else as a solution is the main problem. We do this because we don't realize that we have subconsciously created the "problem" to show ourselves distortions on our lens that need our attention. Once we see the "problem" as the "solution," the negative energy generated by the problem becomes positive energy for the solution.

Here are some ways of laughing at a "problem" until it becomes the "solution," and eventually a miracle:

- If you are a perfectionist, be a perfectionist in your happiness.
- If you have any doubt, doubt the doubt.
- When the world gives you lemons, make lemonade.
- If you are obsessive, obsess about being happy and peaceful.
- If you have "Victimizers," "victimize" your "Victimizers" by turning them into your teachers and love them to death for all they have taught you.

Our "Victimizers" are not the problem. The problem is forgetting to laugh about our beliefs and thoughts about them.

The ability to experience miracles depends on knowing Who We Really Are - as the part of us capable of miracles, and the ability to appreciate all God's Jokes, regardless of how seemingly cruel they may appear.

Dispelling Disease

We may go through our life believing we are, for example, a 45-year-old married, white, female, Catholic, postal worker, who lives in Anytown U.S.A. and has fibromyalgia. We go through life telling everyone that is Who We Are. All those labels are spelled out in words. Those spelled words cast a spell on us, spelling us into the powerful belief systems associated with those labels.

The way we identify ourselves misidentifies us as who we are not and limits our ability to experience miracles.

The first step in liberating ourselves from this identification with the labels we give ourselves is to recognize this as a habit that is a product of our *cult*-ural conditioning from the cult you are a part of. Most people have been so brainwashed into believing they are their thoughts, emotions and all the labels they and others have put on themselves that they don't even consider the True Power they could have if they were to break through the illusions and Powerfully Laugh at it all.

The other option for dispelling disease is by feeling the essence of Who You Are beyond thoughts, beliefs, and emotions, to an awareness beyond any disease. We can recognize the same magical and creative essence that is within us every moment of our life, even while it may appear to be hidden beneath our physical or emotional pain. We can recognize that same magical essence in trees, birds, a chair and in an un-flushed, stinky public bathroom toilet bowl. That essence seems deeply hidden but becomes so obvious once we let go and escape into laughter.

Another way to know Who We Really Are beyond disease, is by knowing who we really are not. We do this every night when we go to sleep. When we are deeply asleep, we forget who we think we are, we forget about diseases and pains, and are more in touch with Who We Really Are. So, as we are falling asleep, we are really waking up more to Who We Really Are, and when we wake up in the morning, we are really falling more asleep to Who We Really Are.

In the same way, when we laugh at our thoughts, we are essentially falling asleep to our thought-based diseased state, and waking up to the healthy state of Who We Really Are.

During deep sleep, people often have delta brainwave frequency. This is a state of consciousness where awareness is detached from personal awareness. This delta frequency can also be a gateway to the Universal Mind and the Collective Unconscious, with a vast landscape of infor-mation that is otherwise unavailable at the conscious level. Awareness of this state can be a gateway to Who We Really Are, and a way to receive Divine messages about how to help cure our disease.

The good news is, we can also get into this healing state during our waking life, but we need to get our ego on our side. This is because many diseases can be caused or worsened by the ego's anger about challenging people and situations. This anger causes a proliferation of toxic biochemicals in our body that predispose to disease. Instead of triggering these toxic biochemicals by engaging in our ego's battle against challenging people, we can get the ego on our side by using a win-win philosophy.

The ego has a need to feel special. Instead of indulging in the parts of ego that thrive on feeling special such as anger, hatred, jealousy, competition, judgments, and fear - we can praise our ego when it finds creative ways of finding unconditional love for all those we most despise (as described in Chapter 13 – in the subsection "Redefine and Shine"). Once we can unconditionally love everyone, we will feel a sense of peace and interconnectedness and reclaim our Wholeness. Then, we will change our biochemistry to one that is healing. Our ego will feel even more special with all these achievements – which encourages our ego to continue helping in this project.

Despite all that we have discussed, we may continue to find it difficult to experience unconditional love for evil people who seem as though they are out to get us, or who have caused serious damage to others or the world. But this continued angst is interfering with our ability to laugh at our thoughts about disease and hence needs correction.

The way to let go of habitual negative thought patterns that cause diseases is to recognize them as habitual thought patterns that have nothing to do with Who We Really Are. Once recognized as such, it is no longer a habitual thought pattern. It becomes a laughter target. Once we recognize and laugh at that pattern enough, it will disappear and our Wholeness and our disease-free consciousness grounded in Who We Really Are will take its place. Rumi said, "Out beyond ideas of wrong-doing and right-doing there is a field. I'll meet you there." That field is the space between our thoughts. It is the space that lies between the stimulus and our habitual response. It is the disease-free place laughter takes us to.

Experiencing Miracles

In summary, a miracle is a wonderful event that is believed to be caused by the power of God. It is also a correction in perception. Since we are created in God's image, to know ourselves is to know God. And since God can create miracles, by knowing Who We Are, we will be more able to see miracles all around us.

The clearer our lens is between the "Light of God" and the mirrors, the more easily God's miracles can be projected onto the Hall of Mirrors.

It is up to us to keep our lens as clean as possible. This can enable us to experience miracles. If our lens is dirty with distortions created by being out of alignment with our authentic self, instead of seeing miracles in our Hall of Mirrors, we will see a world of multiple pathological personalities and traumatic events.

Whenever we see an abnormal personality in the mirror, we can recognize its origin in ourselves and work on this distortion with equanimity, forgiving and loving all those reflections and forgiving ourselves for creating them. Once we do that, we will be aligned with the Light of God, which is perfectly aligned with Who We Really Are.

Another way of getting more in touch with Who *You* Really Are, the *You* capable of miracles, is by no longer basing any aspect of your identity on what you see in the mirrors. This is because Who You Really Are is not who you see in the Hall of Mirrors.

The mirrors give us a good idea of the distortions still needing our attention. Although we no longer derive our identity from the mirrors, it is helpful to use the information gained from them to show us which aspect of the lens would be helpful to "work" on, i.e., laugh about.

During this whole process, we continue laughing at the reflections in the mirrors, appreciating the Inconvenient Joke, finding the jokes hidden in the ironies of our daily life, and seeing the problem as the solution.

Any method that maximally cleans our lens can enhance our ability to experience miracles by correcting our perception. Once you've understood the connections between outer challenges and your ways of thinking, there is an even more advanced process to do. You can also do a deeper cleaning of your lens by noticing the challenges faced by other people - challenges you may not yet have recognized in yourself - and work on these, knowing that if something is in your outer world, it is somewhere in your inner world, within your mind.

For example, if one of your friends is not happy, has an addiction, is greedy, jealous or has any other trait that creates a negative emotional charge in you, you might check to see whether you have a similar trait, whether explicitly manifesting or hiding as a latent tendency. Once identified in someone else, you can focus your attention and correct that latent tendency in yourself.

In this holographic universe, where everything we observe or experience represents aspects of us, by noticing certain aspects of others in ourselves, we can heal them, without waiting for those traits to burst forth and create a mess on our doorstep.

Our erroneous and fixed beliefs may be what has prevented us from experiencing the miracles that Jesus facilitated and told us we are capable of doing.

Whether or not it is possible to help another person heal by healing their challenge within ourselves depends on many factors, including the lessons that need to be learned by the person with the health challenge. Because, although having a health challenge may sound very cruel, it may also be the most loving and compassionate thing our mirrors can do to show us our blockages that need healing if we haven't noticed the gentler messages.

When Jesus said that "I and the Father are one," we can see how this epiphany enabled him to experience miracles. In the context of this book, we could say that his lens was clear and he could experience miracles, because the Light of God was able to shine directly onto his Hall of Mirrors.

Is Everything a Miracle?

Our judgment of what is and is not a miracle may bring us to the realization that there are no miracles, while at the same time, everything is a miracle. If a miracle is a wonderful event which is in some way contrary to our expectations, appears to be unexplainable, and is believed to be caused by the power of God, then there are no miracles. This is because, when searching deeply enough, everything can be explained by lifetimes of distortions in the lens that are seen when the Light of God shines our distortions onto our Hall of Mirrors.

At the same time, everything, including the distorted images, is created by God. Even difficult situations are wonderful events that allow you to see your distortions and clean your lens. So, everything is a miracle.

Our job is to find the hidden jokes and hidden miracles in as many places as we can, using the material world as our props. As Swami Beyondananda says, "The reason we are put in the material world is to get more material." They are presents from God and require being in the "present moment awareness" to find – it takes presence to unwrap our presents. They were placed there by God to make sure you are speaking his language and tuned into His frequency. Once we are tuned in to His frequency, the Jesus version of miracles may be more likely to manifest in our lives.

Greater Miracles than Jesus

One of the most important messages that Jesus delivered is that whoever believes in Him will do the works Jesus has done, and even greater things than these.

As you know, Jesus' miracles included healing diseases, such as paralysis, blindness, deafness, mutism, fever, blood issues, leprosy and restoring a withered hand. Jesus also changed water into wine, walked on water, facilitated the great haul of fishes that fed five thousand people, stilled a storm, caused a fig tree to wither, restored the ear of the high priest's servant, and raised several people from the dead, including Himself.

Once our lens is as perfectly clear as Jesus', the Light of God, capable of miracles, will shine directly onto our Hall of Mirrors. The resulting reflections may have the appearance of, for example, going to the right doctor who performs the most effective procedure, or doing the right hypnosis session that triggers the person with a health challenge to let go of the belief that was causing the illness. They learn whatever they can from that unhealthy personality, and then revert to the one with the normal personality. This may explain how Jesus was able to cure diseases.

We may be able to understand how Jesus created miracles by examining the situation from my allegory. If the world is an illusory Hall of Mirrors, whatever we see is a reflection of our thoughts. Those thoughts make up our "definitions." Whenever we want to change the reflection, we need to look at our definitions that caused that reflection. Unlike the case for Jesus, changing these definitions can be challenging for many people, because their definitions are extremely fixed.

For example, if Jesus' definition of what we call "water" is something solid and can be walked on, and if we wholeheartedly, without a shadow of a doubt, believed in that definition and could be totally oblivious to all the information we may have acquired to the contrary, we may also be able to walk on water. This is the same principle used with bending a spoon.

It is possible that Jesus changed water into wine using the same principles a hypnotist uses to enable people to eat an onion as if it is an apple. Similarly, he may have fed at least five thousand people using hypnotic principles. The power of suggestion may have enabled people to be nourished by a homeopathic quality of food in which the smaller the dose, the more powerful the effects.

Stilling a storm, causing a fig tree to wither, restoring the ear of the high priest's servant and raising several people from the dead, including Himself, etc., may all be possible from our understanding of the Schrodinger's Cat experiment. In this experiment, the cat is theoretically both alive and dead at the same time - until it is observed. Once it is observed, it is either alive or dead. At any moment, there is a storm and no storm, a withered tree and a normal tree, Jesus being alive and dead, etc., each as equal possibilities. In each of those moments, Jesus may have given a powerful "hypnotic suggestion" or used His own clear vision to cause the desired change.

Jesus may have caused the "miraculous" change through a powerful "hypnotic suggestion" or by clarifying His own vision. Each of us may also have this power. As Jesus said, "Whoever believes in me will do the works I have been doing, and they will do even greater things than these."

Wake up Laughing from "Death"

In the *Lazarus Syndrome*, there is a spontaneous return of life after a patient has been declared dead. This syndrome gets its name from Lazarus who, according to the New Testament, was raised from the dead by Jesus.

In the book *Mind-Body Therapy*, hypnotist Thomas Hudson, wrote about the days before embalming when pseudo-death was rather common, explaining, "Chronically ill patients become hyper-suggestible and may mimic all the signs of death when their relatives and medical attendants give up hope."

One young woman had been pronounced dead by six medical attendants 14 days prior to her funeral. "On this day, the little brother, not accepting the reality of her death, cried 'What do you want, sister?' Her mouth moved, asking faintly for water. She revived and lived out a normal span of life[6, 7]."

In the same *Mind-Body Therapy* book, Ernest Rossi describes another case wherein the first spades full of dirt were shoveled onto Roberto Rodriguez's coffin after his heart attack. He suddenly burst open the lid of his coffin, climbed out of his grave, and ran home screaming and swearing. Unfortunately, the shock of seeing the "dead" man burst from the coffin caused his mother-in-law to collapse and die, so she was buried in his place. There are many similar cases of people rising from the "dead[8]."

Since people on the verge of death are hyper-suggestible, in addition to CPR for the body, it can be just as life-saving to give powerful suggestions - CPR for the soul. Such powerful suggestions should be as targeted as possible, perhaps about their children, grandchildren or their unfinished work. Using their first name is important. For example; "Jane, you cannot die! Your children would be lost without you!" Or "Jane, come back, you need to teach the world everything you have learned from your heart attack and your return to life. You can take back control of your body right now! You can do it; I know you can!" All these commands need to be said with an authoritative and forceful tone of voice.

If the "dead" person knows the Powerful Joke, you may even be able to remind them of it. Getting them to laugh at The Joke can encourage them to disassociate from their life challenges instead of from their body. An example would be, "Isn't it funny how you gave yourself a heart attack with all your anger toward (their Frankenstein Monster) when that anger doesn't affect them at all, and the Monster was showing you your blockages to unconditional love?"

Caution: Unless that person has entirely embodied the Joke, don't expect them to be rolling on the floor in fits of laughter. But when used on the right person, once they laugh away their life challenges, they may wake up laughing from "death."

Using any combination of these approaches can sometimes be the catalyst for life-saving "miracles."

Just like Schrodinger's Cat, at each moment, there is the personality that is alive, and one that is dead. Which personality manifests may reflect our beliefs. As Jesus consciously changed his thoughts and vision, everything around him changed in the intended way.

The difference between Jesus and most other people is that Jesus was likely working with a clear lens. When using a clear lens with clear intent, that intent is powerfully manifested. There are none of the interfering distortions seen with people with dissociative identity disorders who can perform apparent haphazard miracles when shifting from one personality to another.

Perhaps this is all possible. But what would doing miracles greater than Jesus look like in today's world?

Does it mean instead of feeding five thousand people, we will have a maître d' serve a banquet to five thousand people at the Ritz Carlton?

Does it mean instead of turning water into wine, we will turn it into Dom Perignon?

Does it mean instead of healing leprosy, we will turn lepers into contestants at the Miss America Beauty Contest?

One way to find out how miracles would manifest through us is by letting go of our fixed beliefs and finding out for ourselves and having fun with the process. This process can take many decades to perfect, so it is helpful to remember that there is never failure, only feedback. Any failures we experience provide us with more information about how to be successful in further attempts. Even if we are never entirely successful in manifesting miracles greater than Jesus', we will certainly be successful in progressively purifying our lens through this process.

Once our lens is clear, we open the space in which miracles happen naturally. Then, instead of being surprised when we see miracles happen, we will be surprised when we don't.

Once we laugh at God's Jokes that appear as major challenges, and allow the laughter to clear our lens of distortions, this laughter becomes infectious. As more people catch the "laughter virus" and figure out the punchline of this grand joke, we may see a major shift within the consciousness of humanity that allows us to experience miracles greater than Jesus'.

Perhaps this global laughter will take humanity to a place beyond thoughts, beyond beliefs and beyond the Illusory World. This laughter might take us to another dimension of reality in which more profound miracles are possible for all. Perhaps that is what Jesus meant by miracles greater than His.

But just as Jesus faced the Great Abyss through His crucifixion, perhaps for us to be free of The Illusion and eventually experience miracles greater than His, we must continue on our Hero's Journey into our own Great Abyss.

"If you stay in the center and embrace death with your whole heart, you will endure forever."

— Lao-Tzu

Chapter Seventeen
Dying to Wake Up

Warning: This chapter contains some graphic information about death. Readers who are going through challenging times or are depressed, emotionally unstable, or have any other psychological or emotional condition should skip this entire chapter. If this applies to you, please seek support via friends, family and/or Lifeline and professional services.

Many people who have had near-death experiences are transformed by them. Wouldn't it be great to have this transformation without needing to die? Let's look at how this may be possible and how we can have the benefits of dying without dying.

Lao Tzu said: "If you want to be reborn, let yourself die." Spiritual sages have exhorted seekers of truth to, "Die before you die." This process of experiencing the world beyond the Illusory World required my dying to conditioned thoughts during my Vipassana epiphany and my near-death experience in the sweat lodge. I realized that, in order to know how to live a life beyond the Illusory World, I had to surrender to the Great Abyss.

Death is the ultimate annihilation of not just the body, but the ego. Once our ego has been annihilated through a "death" in our lives, we are never the same. The annihilation of the ego allows us to be free of the Illusory World and allows the Light of God to shine directly onto our Hall of Mirrors and manifest all the miracles that come along with that Light. One not so tiny problem - once we physically die, there is no one home to experience these miracles. The solution, therefore, is to die before our death.

The way we die before our death is by making peace with the varying degrees of death of the ego we face on an ongoing basis. We do this by facing the Abysses of our daily life. This facing, and then surrendering to the Abyss helps in the annihilation of the ego.

This surrender can take the form of a loss of a job, loss of a relationship, loss of a loved one, a dire health diagnosis, facing poverty, etc. It can also take on more subtle forms of suffering that can nevertheless fluff up our ego defenses – irritations like getting cut off in traffic, dealing with a rude salesperson, or getting one's hair rearranged by God in the wind and rain. These are examples of the small Abysses of death we face daily. These opportunities give us the choice of resisting or accepting the situation. They involve either suffering or dying to our conditioned thoughts - through laughter.

These difficult situations are invitations to enter the Great Abyss in varying degrees. If we resist these invitations, we create more distortions on our lens and shape the future potential of facing more challenging opportunities to learn the lessons we've resisted. If we surrender and accept life on life's terms, we enter a deeper level of The Zone and emerge more empowered to respond to similar challenges. Eventually those challenges won't be reflecting in our mirrors, because we'll have let go of the worry or anger and shifted into higher realms of personal and global awareness. The more we are able to welcome the Abyss as learning opportunities, the higher we go on our Emotional Scale.

There is only one problem with welcoming the Great Abyss - our ego does not go along with the plan. Our ego has a tremendous fear of annihilation. This fear contributes to our subconscious fear of death that we carry with us wherever we go.

The ego resists its annihilation in a multitude of ways. It believes we'd be unhappy waking up to Who We Really Are - a place in which there is no ego. The problem is, the more we wish to annihilate the ego, the more fear we experience. The more fear we experience, the more we listen to the ego because it speaks the loudest. And if that wasn't challenging enough, there's another culprit that is in on the plot to keep us from living in The Zone.

So the plot thickens… Not only is the *ego* guarding against our escape from our illusion of mirrors, but so is the *super-ego*. The super-ego is the part of our mind that judges the ego and the spiritual path of others. It guides us to be holier than thou, and judges others for their heathenistic practices that are always inferior to ours. An extreme example of those with a highly developed super-ego is the "pious" people who have killed millions of people in the name of God, through "Holy Wars."

Prisoners of Our Own Mind

In a plot twist, it turns out that the part of our mind that we trust the most, the morally superior super-ego, turns out to be a double agent. It seems so spiritual on the surface, but because we trust in it, it can be even more diabolical than the ego. This trust may be misplaced because the super-ego, like the ego, has a vested interest in keeping us a prisoner to the Illusory World.

For all these years we've entrusted our super-ego with helping us escape the Illusory World through our religious and spiritual practices while at the same time the super-ego may be another security guard at the exit door from The Illusion.

Both the ego and super-ego prevent our exit from The Illusion because their survival depends on keeping alive this delusion that we are our thoughts and our body. They are deathly afraid of letting go of this delusory belief that fuels their very existence. Even though our freedom lies in letting go of these beliefs, the ego and super-ego distrust this freedom and do their very best to make sure we never escape.

The plot thickens even more because not only are the ego and super-ego guarding against our escape, they are joined at the exits by our Frankenstein Monsters.

There is a particular Frankenstein Monster that is the scariest one of them all, and it is guarding the master exit. This Master Monster is composed of our fear of death; it is composed of our fear that we will be de-composed.

Death is the Master Monster because many of our other fears are a re-sult of our fear of death. Our fear of death is therefore the Monster of Monsters, the deeper cause of most of our other fears.

The reason these Monsters are so masterful is they work through stealth technology, at the unconscious level. Because we see other "nor-mal" people also believing they are a victim of a cruel world, we are not even aware we are a prisoner of this Illusory World. Since we don't realize we are its prisoner, we don't even bother looking for a way out. We con-tinue believing we are a victim of a cruel God because we don't see the world as a gallery of mirrors.

Just when we think the plot is as thick as it can get, it thickens even more. Trying to escape The Illusion through death is not the answer be-cause the security around the Hall of Mirrors is so extreme that very few people in history have escaped it.

The reason the security is so high is because until we learn all the les-sons from the distortions on our lens, our distorted Hall of Mirrors will follow us wherever we go, lifetime after lifetime - because it is a product of our mind.

Having had those brief glimpses of the world on the other side of the Illusory World during my ten-day meditation and near-death experience, I realize how much I am a prisoner of The Illusion.

Although our ego and super-ego seem to be complicating our exit, they are just doing their best in their assigned roles. They are there to pro-tect us from a cruel world. They were born out of fear to protect us from those enemies that were perceived to be outside of us, not realizing those enemies are really our shadows.

These bodyguards may be standing guard in the background as you read this book, skeptical of this laughter, fearful it will cause you to lay down your guard and become a victim of a cruel world.

The skepticism of the ego and super-ego is the reason for all the other strategies discussed throughout the book. If laughter at the Powerful Joke and at our thoughts were all it took, we would all be laughing Buddhas by now.

Laughing Our Way Home

The process of forgetting to laugh didn't arise overnight. **The process of learning to laugh is much more complicated than the process of forgetting because of the strength of the ego and super-ego, the accumulation of distortions, and the ever-strengthening habit of forgetting to laugh.** But this process of learning to laugh can be expedited by carefully reading and perhaps re-reading this book.

It is important to remember that the ego and super-ego, and your Frankenstein Monsters, are not your enemies. They are there to help you. They want you to be safe and happy. They just each have different ways of achieving this goal.

Since their birth, at the time you forgot to laugh and began developing fears, they were each doing the best they could.

As you read this material and gradually experiment with some of the suggestions, I hope that you, your ego and super-ego may all find that laughter is not only safe, it is a fun way to enter The Zone. Since they all want the very best for you, once you all notice that you can achieve much better results without their help, they will realize they can either take an early retirement or take on a new job of helping you laugh.

In order to demonstrate to them that all is well, from time to time we may need to face the Abyss once more, where our fear of death is ignited. Embracing and laughing at our fear of death can be extremely helpful in order to wholeheartedly laugh at The Joke in a way that demonstrates to our ego and super-ego that all is well.

Advising a child to laugh at their thoughts of death may be all that is needed because their egos haven't developed masses of fearful information about it. As adults, if we were to simply laugh at all the thoughts that create our fear of death, our egos would mount a major revolt.

Even though Lao Tzu was absolutely right in saying, "As soon as you have made a thought, laugh at it," this is often much easier said than done.

If it is too difficult for you to do as Lao Tzu recommends and laugh at every thought as it arises, a paradoxical path is to totally disregard his teaching and do just the opposite. Allow your thoughts to run wild and stalk your thoughts about death. Once you truly see, examine, explore, and understand your erroneous beliefs about death, you will feel more comfortable with death, and therefore with life.

Although death may be very frightening to most of us, many people celebrate it. Ecclesiastes 7:1 says, "The day of death is better than one's day of birth." On her deathbed, Teresa of Avila rejoiced, "The hour I have long wished for is now come." Many Orthodox Hassidic Jews celebrate death. Other cultures celebrate when a loved one dies because they know they are going to a better place.

In our culture, death can seem very frightening due to our cultural conditioning that often includes specified periods of mourning to wear black and grieve.

Some people resist life and wish to die to escape their distorted mirror reflections. If they get their wish, everything they resisted in this life will likely show up in different and more challenging ways in their next life until they learn the lessons necessary to clear their lens.

Whatever we resist - whether it is an abusive spouse, an arrogant teenager, needing to pay bills with money we don't have, facing memories from childhood, paying taxes to a seemingly corrupt government, or facing death - all these resistances are personally designed to show us our blockages to the Light of God. Once we laugh away all these blockages and laugh in the face of death, the Light of God shines directly on our Hall of Mirrors, and we return to our real home - Heaven on Earth.

Laughing at Death

Lao Tzu said, "If you stay in the center and embrace death with your whole heart, you will endure forever." When we embrace anything we resisted, we take another step into the Abyss and another step closer to The Zone.

Facing our fear of death is like my experience of facing the pain during my meditation retreat as well as anytime we face The Great Abyss. The more we fear and resist pain and death, or any other Abyss, the more suffering we experience. The more we get to know the truth about pain, death and every other Abyss at the deepest level - and discover that everything is just temporarily arising and then passing away - the more peaceful we will feel. This is because, as I learned from my meditation experience with severe pain, the core essence of everything is the core essence of God: Peace, and Light.

We know that for many of us, death arises and passes away. Through hypnosis studies, we can be reasonably certain about some version of reincarnation. In a hypnotic state, many subjects have been able to recall details from a previous life - details they couldn't possibly have known if they hadn't been reincarnated.

Although it may sometimes be helpful to have a fear of death to help keep us alive and inspire us to avoid dangerous situations, fear is a product of distorted thought. Thoughts often prevent people from being in The Zone where they can function at their peak. In a thought-free state, miracles become possible. Such was the case with Angela Cavallo, who lifted a Chevy Impala, under which her son was pinned. Lydia Angiyou saved a child by fighting off a polar bear. If either of these women had any fearful thoughts about the situation or any doubts about their capabilities, they likely wouldn't have achieved those miracles. Even in emergency situations, fear is not always our friend. I had a huge fear of death until my near-death experience in which I experienced an extremely Blissful surrender. Until then, pain and death were among the two things I most resisted. After experiences of extreme Bliss with the things I most resisted, my perspective has dramatically changed.

Just as discovering the truth beyond fears about pain and death was helpful for me, discovering the truth about death may be helpful to you. Then you can decide for yourself the degree of fear that is right for you.

As we begin to stalk death or any Abyss, we begin to notice where our thoughts are profoundly out of alignment with the Light of God and out of alignment with the absolute truth of the situation. Just as late-night comedians have discovered regarding corrupt politicians, the greater the corruption, the greater the opportunity for laughter. Any misalignment with the truth causes a painful "truth-ache." This often leads to distortions, which over time leads to a plaque build-up on our lens. This build-up eventually leads to truth-decay and regardless of the time on your watch, it will always feel like tooth-hurty.

Truth is the solution to finding freedom in the world beyond illusions. Jesus said, "And you will know the truth, and the truth will set you free." By setting us free with this message, Jesus is our truth fairy.

There is a story of a gunman who broke into a car with his finger on the trigger of a handgun, ready to fire it at a woman. The woman calmly turned around and said, "Go ahead and shoot me, and I'll go straight to Heaven, and you'll go straight to Hell."

Truth extraction can evoke fear and hit a nerve which can be extremely painful. To prevent this, we need to use mental-floss and laugh away the lies, so we can avoid truth-decay and not need any drugs whatsoever. Once we wake up laughing without medication - we will be in a state of transcend-dental-medication.

Unleashing the Wizard Within

Learning more truth about the nature of death was of vital importance to overcoming my fear about it.

We can look at the fear of death as something being controlled by a little man (our thoughts) working behind the scenes (in our subconscious mind), much like the Wizard of Oz. Its job is to create fearful thoughts and images (our Frankenstein Monsters). All it takes is a Toto (laughter) to pull back the curtain and expose the truth behind the great and powerful Wizard. Once we discover that all those fearful images were created by the Wizard behind the curtain (our thoughts), we will automatically laugh away our fearful images (click our heels three times saying "There's no place like home") and the fearful game is over.

The funny part of this joke is that the Wizard behind the curtain is essentially none other than you! You are that little wizard behind the curtain creating all those fearful thoughts which are creating all those fearful emotions that are scaring the bejeebers out of you.

You can use this Wizard of Oz analogy for your fear of death or any other confrontation with the Great Abyss you may experience as you progress on your Hero's Journey.

Now that you know how to pull back the curtain on the Wizard of Oz, let's look at the benefits of doing so.

If you know anyone who has had a near-death experience, you will know that many of them are transformed. They lose their fear of death, become more spiritual, and engage in more philosophical and abstract thinking. They are less competitive and have a new life purpose. They have more psychic abilities and expansive concepts of love, as well as a child-like sense of curiosity, wonder, and joy. They appreciate the Powerful Joke, even when it appears to be Inconvenient. Once they laugh at the Joke, their *laugh* force nourishes their *life* force.

Our fear of death depletes our life force. That fear is so deeply repressed that we are often not even aware of it. It is only when we get older that we begin to acknowledge it.

But why wait? Now is the time to eliminate our fear of death. We do that and take back our life force by laughing at The Illusion.

Most people are not quite ready to lighten up about death. Death can seem very frightening. Death can seem darker than dark, but it is a perfect darkness. Without that perfect darkness in the night sky, we wouldn't be able to appreciate the perfect light of the stars. The darker the dark, the more brilliant the stars. With more rain comes more rainbows.

When Jesus said, "The truth will set you free," I believe he meant that truth can result in freedom from everything, including frustrations over a corrupt government and our other "Victimizers," as well as our fear of death.

Another reason we are not ready to lighten up about death is that we fear the unknown. As we look further into the nature of death, it won't be so frightening.

Repeated Warning: Because the following section contains graphic information about death, readers who are going through challenging times, feeling depressed or emotionally unstable in any way should skip the remainder of this chapter.

The Inspiration Gained from Expiration

Before my near-death experience, I had a huge fear of death. I eventually realized that the subconscious fear of death was always in the background, keeping me from feeling completely free and alive. With this understanding, I wanted to experience my virtual death while I was still alive and get it out of the way. I saw how most of the fears in my life were a consequence of my underlying fear of death. I was hopeful that once I experienced my virtual death, my ego would die in the process, and I would have a greater experience of Who I Really Am while I was still alive.

I also realized that my subconscious fear of death may be worse than actually dying.

Here are some things I did that you may wish to do as well:

- I wrote a letter to a loved one who had died. I told them how I felt about their death. I listed all the feelings their death brought up for me. During this process, I felt all the pain and embraced it completely, and without judgment. I explored the pain surrounding death while avoiding adding any unnecessary mental commentaries or creating additional mental stories that lead to more suffering.
- I made a list of what I would do if I only had four months to live.
- I uncovered my irrational beliefs about death, including the idea that if I didn't think or talk about death, maybe it wouldn't happen, or that it's the end of the road, or that it's the ultimate sign of failure, all of which are not true.
- I wrote my own eulogy. I emphasized all my positive attributes and listed all my accomplishments. I visualized telling everyone

they could allow themselves to fully release all their emotions about my death in every way they can, by crying, screaming, or swearing at God. I chose a song that reflected my life ("Imagine" by John Lennon), to be sung just before the completion of the service.

It was healing to accept the inevitability of my death and immerse myself in the dying process while embracing all my emotions. It seemed helpful to fully let go and surrender to the grief this brought up. I allowed my emotions to be completely expressed, and released.

I also visited my brother's grave and spoke with his spirit. These exercises were all grave undertakings.

Warning: *If you have found these exercises challenging, please skip to the end of this chapter.*

I also did a self-guided meditation on my own death which was something like this:

I shifted into a relaxed state, in a quiet and comfortable place, and closed my eyes. Once I was relaxed, I visualized myself sitting deep within a peaceful forest. Dappled light cast sparkles on richly colored leaves. The trees swayed gently in the soothing breeze. A bird sang a light, happy song. A beautiful nearby waterfall complemented the sound of softly rustling leaves.

As I looked down from the other end of the forest onto a gravesite, I saw people quietly gathering near a clearing. I sensed something special was about to happen. I noticed that these people were my friends and family and they were all dressed in black. They seemed very sad, and some were crying.

After a few minutes, my best friend arrived and made his way to the podium where he began speaking about a very dear person who had died. He said a few words about that person's qualities and personality, and as he went on, I realized he was speaking about me. He choked up as he was overcome with sadness, and tears poured down his face.

Several minutes later, I saw a coffin carried by four close friends who were also dressed in black. They looked as if they were in a state of shock. I realized this coffin contained my own dead body. They carried the coffin to the gravesite, and I saw it lowered into a deep hole in the ground. Once the coffin had reached its final resting place, I allowed my awareness to shift to the inside of the coffin.

I imagined hearing the thump of dirt on my casket and realized they were going to be the last sounds I would ever hear. I smelled the clean, moist soil surrounding my coffin and sensed my body immersed in a darkness so thick that I could almost cut it with a knife.

I was ready to go. I mentally said goodbye to all my loved ones for the very last time. I got deeply in touch with my emotions, and those of my friends and family, as the finality of what was happening suddenly struck me at my core. This would be the place my body would remain for all of eternity.

I would never smell anything other than the smell of this dirt, which would surround my body for eternity. I would never hear anything other than this absolute silence nor see anything other than this absolute darkness. With this realization, I experienced waves of profound sadness.

I got in touch with my feelings as I mourned the end of my life on earth. I'd felt all the emotions arising as I said goodbye to my loved ones for the very last time. Now, I allowed my body to be totally taken over by sadness and grief, as I mourned the loss of everything I ever possessed and all my hopes for a better future in this lifetime. I allowed every emotion to become fully alive and expressed. After a few minutes, I felt the emotions receding like waves from the shore, little by little, until no emotion remained.

I felt more peaceful than I had ever felt before. I laughed as I realized that this experience was what I had feared my whole life. It was such a relief to get it out of the way, so I could now live the rest of my life without that underlying fear.

I stayed immersed in that peace. I felt around to get to know the part of me that remained. It was the part of me that had always been there, immortal, and one with God. I realized that this is Who I Really Am. I stayed with this feeling for a while.......

As I looked back at my life, I reviewed and registered everything I had learned over the course of my life. I also saw what lessons I still wished to learn and the situations and people I wanted to learn from for the remainder of my life.

I took that experience with me as I slowly opened my eyes and looked around me with a fresh outlook. I began experiencing life anew, as though I was reborn and seeing everything for the first time.

Note: If you skipped ahead, you can resume from here.

As I imagined my own death, I was bawling my eyes out about how overwhelmingly sad it was to experience myself from inside the casket. Saying goodbye to my friends and family was extremely difficult for me, believing I would never see them again. But once I surrendered my ego attachment to everything, I felt a tremendous sense of peace.

I found that dying felt about as stressful as changing my clothes or changing television stations. I would not like to spend lifetime after lifetime watching the same channel on television or wearing the same clothes. After a while I would be bored and exchange my old tattered clothes for brand new ones. After this experience, my compulsion to have the same body forever seemed more like a habit than a preference. Indeed, continuing to inhabit the same body can be "in-habit forming."

But if I knew that a new body would bring me the lessons and experiences I needed, I'd want to choose that body and life situation for my next life.

As I synthesized my experiences, I realized that facing any Great Abyss in a state of peace and equanimity is absolutely necessary - or a similar challenge will show up on my doorstep very soon. We can face this Abyss with whatever works best for us. For me, laughter works best, though it is still a work in progress.

We basically have three options for facing the Great Abyss. We can embrace and heal our relationship with each Abyss experience during this lifetime or during our next lifetime, or we can save ourselves a lot of suffering by helping to heal them all during this lifetime through LaughGnosis, meditation techniques, or other modalities and practices.

I had an enormous fear of death until I experienced my own near-death experience in the sweat lodge, and my Vipassana experience of having no thoughts, which I came to see as the death of the ego. Once I had these experiences, I felt much more relaxed about death.

I found it very interesting how, in my imagined funeral, people responded to my death by being overcome with sadness, as though I was suffering. In my imagined reality, it was just the opposite. My virtual death resulted in a state of bliss.

This blissful state may be experienced by some people who go through a natural death.

However, although there is as of yet no way to research hard data on this, it is generally thought that the experience beyond death may be very different for someone who commits suicide to escape their life situation. In their next life, they may be faced with even more extreme versions of the lessons they tried to escape in this lifetime. Someone who commits suicide may appear to have gotten over their fear of death. Suicide however, is the ultimate resistance to the present moment, and therefore creates the largest distortions in their lens. This brings forth another array of extremely frightening Frankenstein Monsters. Until the traveling soul stops resisting, starts accepting, and finds its way to experiencing peace with its projected Monsters, it will continue to encounter these aberrations from lifetime to lifetime. Wherever it goes, its holographic world will follow, complete with all the lessons it needs to learn.

Now that I had made peace with the Great Abyss of death, I felt ready to be reborn, feeling that I'd been given the opportunity to live a second time. I felt willing to let go of the ego-based ways I saw reality, and instead embraced my life's purpose from a more cooperative and loving perspective, full of child-like curiosity, wonder, and joy.

Although I had many great realizations, I must admit that putting them into practice and not getting triggered by facing yet another Great Abyss remains a challenge. There remains a great division between what I knew and what I've practiced. Remembering to laugh at God's jokes through all the twists and turns of writing this book helped me dramatically with this process.

By remembering to laugh at God's hidden jokes, I learned a few more things about facing death. One thing I learned was that fear of death and fear of any Abyss I may encounter, regardless of the form it may take, is just an illusion created by thoughts I forgot to laugh at. The best way to learn about death is by imagining myself laughing from my casket..........from the *insight*-out.

I had gone through my whole life fearing death, never realizing that fear was in the back of my mind. This unconscious fear had prevented me from thoroughly enjoying my life and living in The Zone. Now that I know that the death of the eternal essence of Who I Really Am is not possible, what is there to take so seriously? Since the world is an illusion, what can die other than the **ego's** conditioned thought system that generated this Illusory World? Would you prefer to transcend the ego's thought system by physically dying to it, and facing the possibility of greater challenges in your next lifetime; or would you prefer laughing your way out of the ego's Illusory World to live in a Heaven on Earth, and encourage others to do the same?

I also learned that getting comfortable with my expiration is a great inspiration. Hopefully I will inspire many others to enjoy this inspiration before their expiration.

As this chapter neared completion and I was eating an egg from breakfast, I also realized that the secret of true inner peace is digesting.

Although many people would agree that eating is great, few would agree that digesting is the secret to true inner peace. Just to clarify - I said nothing about food. I said the secret of true inner peace is *die-jesting*.

Since we now know that death is not to be feared, let's die-jesting! And since all there is is the present moment, let's start jesting now!

As I contemplated this egg as a hologram of the Universe, I received its message and remembered how important it is to wake up laughing at the Powerful yoke, knowing that if I don't laugh, the yoke's on me.

I also realized that when I die-jesting, this will increase the chance of "laugh after death."

"Heaven is here - you just have to know how to live it. And Hell too is here, and you know perfectly well how to live it. It is only a question of changing your perspective."

— Osho

Chapter Eighteen
Finding Heaven on Earth

We have now let go of important blockages to our Authentic Laughter through forgiveness, unconditional love, knowing Who We Really Are and the true nature of reality. We have even made peace with death. We are now ready to use these tools to help find our authentic laughter to help us experience Heaven on Earth.

The truth is, it is not necessary to do any of those things in order to find Heaven. Heaven can be a path more than a goal. The more we strive to get to Heaven, the further away we may go, if that striving is coming from a resistance to where we are right now. The Heavenly experience of smelling the flowers along our path is where Heaven already is. The joke is that once we give up the search for Heaven, we realize we are already Here.

Heaven, health, and miracles are all around us once we know how to find them.

The wizard within us created all sorts of Frankenstein Monsters, devils, and Luciferians to reflect our fears. We made our reflections look as frightening as possible to scare ourselves awake. Now, it is up to us to use these Monsters as fuel for our authentic laughter.

Although Luciferians may appear evil, as you know, in the yin/yang symbol, within the white half of the symbol is a small black circle. And within the black half is a small white circle.

Within the darkest of the dark, there is always light. It is because of the darkest of dark skies that we can fully appreciate a bright star. It is up to us to find that bright star within the darkness of global chaos and political corruption, the goodness within evil, the laughter within sadness, and the angel within the devil. **Then, we can find Heaven wherever we go.**

This may be a difficult process – to find the angels within the demons or ghouls when some days it's hard enough to find our car keys. But those dark entities can be our greatest teachers. After all.........demons are a ghoul's best friend.

The challenge is to find unconditional love for Hitler, and even to find this love for Lucifer. Finding unconditional love for Lucifer may seem very demeaning if we don't know de-meaning of Lucifer. Although commonly used as a name of the devil, Lucifer is a Latin word that literally means "light bringer" or "light bearer." Lux, luci means "light," and "fer" means "bear" or "carry." The meaning of Lucifer as "light bearer" is an appropriate name, once we understand that the greatest oppressors can be our greatest pathways to light.

We've spent most of our lives focusing on our Frankenstein Monsters as though they were evil. These Monsters caused us to focus on the black part of the yin/yang symbol so intensely that we didn't notice the white circle within it.

Our Frankenstein Monsters are essentially playing a game with us. They are chasing us across the giant yin/yang game board of our life until we find the small white circle within the big black half.

That small white circle is the key to laughing at the Inconvenient Joke. It is the Bliss within the pain, the God Essence within all the Luciferians in the world, and every Inconvenient Joke within the world we see. Once we find this small white circle and live our lives within it, we will see Heaven in all the evil in our world.

Even though we are talking about evil Luciferians, it is helpful to continually remind ourselves that Luciferians are light bearers. They are here to encourage us to find the light within the darkness.

They are doing this by pushing all our buttons until we dig deeply enough to find the Powerful humor within their "Jokes" that seem so horrifying and inconvenient to laugh at. Perhaps that is the main reason for their existence.

Nevertheless, as Albert Einstein said, "God doesn't play dice with the Universe." If those Frankenstein Monsters and Hitlers were not necessary to help us find inner peace, they wouldn't be in our lives. They are there to show us the distortions on our lens that are blocking our deep peace. Once we can laugh at the Inconvenient Joke, we will see how these "evil" Luciferians are here to help us see the deep perfection within everything.

We can think of the small white circle within the black part of the yin/yang symbol as a white rabbit hole. The Luciferians are causing these major challenges in the world to challenge us to go deeper into that white rabbit hole. The deeper down the rabbit hole we go, the more we will begin to recognize the perfection in everything.

Because it is difficult to describe in words how to go deeply down into the rabbit hole, let's review how we got so far out of the rabbit hole in the first place. This should help clarify how to get back down into its depths. Let's begin this journey by reviewing one version of a story that happened a long time ago in the Garden of Eden.

Trading Heaven for Knowledge

Adam and Eve were living in a state of Bliss and perfect Nirvana in the Heavenly Garden of Eden. God told them that they could eat from any tree except from the Tree of The Knowledge of Good and Evil. If they ate from that tree, they would surely die.

One day, a snake came to Eve and told her to eat from the Tree of Knowledge to become smart like God. Eve told the snake that God told them never to eat from that tree because if they did, they would surely die. The snake responded that everything God told her about dying is a lie and the apple from that tree would make her wise like God.

Believing the snake, Eve ate an apple from the Tree of Knowledge and gave some of it to Adam.

The fruit did not make Adam and Eve wise like God, but they did realize for the first time that they were naked. They were embarrassed and made skirts of fig leaves.

Eating from the Tree of Knowledge is considered to be the original sin. Suddenly, Adam and Eve needed to hide themselves with fig leaves because they felt embarrassed, believing there were others outside of them who were different from them, judging them – others with whom they were not connected at the deepest level. This represents the origin of the stepping out of the peaceful, blissful non-local mind, and stepping into the illusion of separation and dualistic thinking. This false knowledge takes us out of alignment with the truth of our non-locality and opens the door to subsequent suffering.

Although Eve gets a lot of flak for eating from that tree, Knowledge can be wonderful, as long as we continue searching for Who We Really Are - beyond the limitations of worldly knowledge. If we allow knowledge to make us believe that who we are is affected by any of this "knowledge," we will have "no-ledge" over a bottomless pit of suffering.

Eating from the apple of limited knowledge essentially gave rise to the Hall of Mirrors. Before eating the apple, man was perfectly aligned with the Light of God. The belief in separation caused by eating the apple was responsible for the distortion in the lens and distorted reflections in the mirrors.

Before eating the apple, they felt united with all of creation. There was no need to challenging people or situations to help them find their authentic selves. They were perfectly aligned with the Light of God and able to manifest all of their heart's desires. Because of this, there were no cravings, no aversions, and no suffering. All there was, was the experience of living in The Zone in perfect unity, and the perfect experience of Heaven on Earth.

From eating the apple and the subsequent sex between Adam and Eve arose all of humanity, and all the associated suffering resulting from being human. Eating the apple resulted in the realization of their nakedness. This may have caused them to feel embarrassed, and no longer at ease; thereby creating the first, ongoing, sexually transmitted dis-ease.

No Thanks! Trading Knowledge Back for Heaven

The way to eat from a tree of higher knowledge and find Heaven on Earth is by recognizing that all our Frankenstein Monsters and all the violence in the world are a reflection of our mind. It is helpful to see everything going on in the world and know that, on some deep level, it is reflecting what is going on in our mind. This is the Universal Law: "As within, so without." This law suggests that we are 100% responsible for everything going on in our world, as difficult as that idea can be to digest.

Our job is to see the truth of that, to experience the disgust of that, to let go of all our judgments of that, and then to finally laugh at that.

Taking personal responsibility for all the evils in our world may seem like an extremely masochistic task. But as we continue the process, instead of feeling as though we are taking the blame for all the problems in the world, we feel empowered beyond what we ever had imagined possible. Because if we were are to take 100% of the blame, then we need to take 100% of the credit when we see the positive changes in our reflections after we make the powerful changes in ourselves. The snake is the key to understanding how the Illusory World of Hell began. The snake was re-sponsible for the original sin that caused us to forget our experience of Heaven, living in a collective soup of Consciousness that is perfectly Whole and aligned with the Light of God. We can think of the snake as the enlisting agent of The Illusion that caused us to be its prisoner, while it was working as a *Civil Serpent.*

By continuing to forget to laugh at the possibility that separation is even possible, we are essentially continuing to take small bites of that apple every moment of our lives. In so doing, we become increasingly possessed by the belief in separation. The exercises that will be discussed in the next chapter are designed to help exorcize that diabolical belief.

Based on my experiences and research, one way to reclaim Heaven is by laughing at, forgiving and unconditionally loving all the Frankenstein Monsters and all the snakes in our life. Once we fully appreciate all their teachings and see them as our portal into the depths of the rabbit hole to

Heaven, they can take us to the most fabulous experience of Heaven on Earth.

Once we wholeheartedly laugh at all dualistic thoughts and laugh at the possibility of living anywhere other than Heaven, we reclaim our place within the collective soup of Consciousness, free to experience Heaven wherever we go.

Choosing the small white circle of the yin/yang, the positive interpretation within perceived negativity, leads us down the rabbit hole to Heaven. It is in the "rabbit hole" that we find our "Hole-ness." That hole leads to the depths of our Oneness with God – a Oneness that was waiting for us all along.

"Out of difficulties grow miracles. "
— Jean de la Bruyere

Chapter Nineteen
Changing Faults into Laughter

Now that we know some of the major barriers to laughter, let's talk about ways to incorporate it into our daily life.

The main challenge we face with experiencing laughter is that we often forget how to find our authentic laugh. One way to find this authentic laugh is by remembering our FAULTS.

FAULTS is a mnemonic for *Forgiveness, Awareness, Unconditional love, Laughter, Thanks*, and *Smile*. In order to authentically laugh at the Inconvenient Joke, it is necessary to Forgive, have Awareness and Unconditional love, Laugh and give Thanks.

You should have a good appreciation for the power of Forgiveness and Unconditional love from previous chapters, so let's talk about Awareness, Thanks, Smile, and Laughter.

Awareness

Awareness is being aware of Who We Really Are. In this awareness, there is the dissolution of conditioned thoughts. There is an acceptance of everything exactly as it is. There is no craving for anything to be different, nor an aversion to anything as it is. Pure awareness gives us the ability to perceive things, people, places and situations exactly as they are, bypassing the filters of our conditioned thoughts. Within a state of heightened awareness, we live in The Zone.

Because laughing at our thoughts and at The Powerful Joke helps us helps clear away conditioned thoughts, it helps us attain the state of pure awareness and enter The Zone. Once we are in The Zone, we are aware of more of the Jokes all around us. As we become more aware of the Jokes all around us, this propels us deeper into The Zone. This drives us into a vicious cycle of ever-growing awareness and expansion into the higher levels of The Zone.

We more easily live in The Zone when we have no craving for things to be different. It is okay to have preferences, and okay to have a preference to have no cravings. The main difference between having a craving and having a preference is that having a preference means being attached to the outcome. Even when we may prefer things to be different, there is no craving for them to be different, nor an aversion to them remaining as they are.

Having no cravings is helpful because, as we can see from our life, cravings and aversions can seem like bottomless pits - and cause a lot of internal turmoil and suffering, especially when they are not fulfilled according to our desires.

If a person is being abused, even if that abuse may reflect distortions in their lens, they still take appropriate actions and don't just sit around laughing about it. The difference for one who has awareness is that their actions flow from a place of Deep Inner Peace. The more we can be in The Zone, the more effective we will be in whatever we do.

Some people believe that they need the fuel of anger to make them stronger and more effective. But an archer knows that if they feel anxiety or any other emotion that distracts their focus, they will be unable to hit their target. Professional boxers make it a policy not to become *angry* with their opponent. Although one would think that anger at their opponent would help them win the match, they find that anger interferes with their ability to stay in The Zone, the state of awareness where they are most effective.

Have you ever taken a test when you were nervous or upset about something and couldn't recall the answers? Have you noticed how some answers just come to you when you are relaxed, like in the shower? The question is, how do we take that state of The Zone with us wherever we go?

Living in The Zone in Our Daily Life

The ability to remain in a heightened state of awareness, living in The Zone, in our daily life can be easy when having dinner with our beloved partner. It can be more difficult to access as we are exposed to progressively more challenging situations, unless we turn the whole paradigm around and start to use these challenges to help us go deeper into The Zone, using the pain to get to Bliss, as I discovered during those many hours of painful sitting during the ten-day meditation retreat.

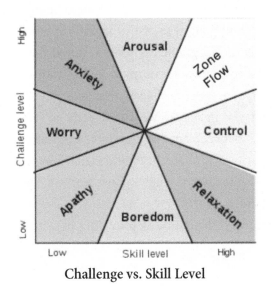

Challenge vs. Skill Level

This graph above shows that the enormous global challenges we are facing are providing us with the perfect backdrop to demonstrate the skills we have acquired over the years to propel us deeper into the "The Zone/Flow."

As we look around our world, it is easy to blame others for all our problems. But what if they are providing us with these very challenging times to push us out of anxiety, apathy, boredom, and worry to get us as deeply as possible into the top right corner of the chart above, "The Zone/heightened state of awareness/Flow.

Some people believe that Earth is a planet for the immature soul when, indeed, the opposite is likely the case. We are the chosen ones - faced with global challenges that are providing us with the ideal fuel to go into depths of The Zone/heightened state of awareness/Flow, that was not possible in previous generations.

This may be an ideal time in human evolution to become an Ascended Master. There have not been many times in known history when such a wealth of spiritual and scientific knowledge was widely available at the click of a button, against the backdrop of such intense global challenges to the extreme level that they threaten the survival of humanity. This is the ideal combination to propel us as deeply as possible into the right upper corner of this graph. We have acquired the skills necessary to face these challenges. Now it's time to demonstrate our integration of these skills, to attain new peaks of awareness.

If not for today's challenges, we would likely be vacillating at the bottom of the chart - between apathy, boredom, and relaxation. If we didn't have the necessary skills to see beyond the illusions and if we took our thoughts seriously instead of laughing at them, we would be vacillating between worry and anxiety.

Today's unique combination is providing us with the rocket fuel to blast off well past the right upper corner of this graph - toward infinity. This is helping us get closer toward God consciousness. **Instead of being angry about all our challenges, let's celebrate them for helping us access the depths of The Zone! Once we use all our skills to face these challenges, there will no longer be a need for our scary reflections, and they will likely miraculously disappear.**

Living in a heightened state of awareness is living in a state in which excitement intersects with equanimity.

Living in a heightened state of awareness in The Zone is like being in the eye of the hurricane that we ride during the chaotic storms of our daily life.

For some people, living in a heightened state of awareness in The Zone happens more rapidly than for others. Those who find it more challenging may benefit from LaughGnosis. People who access The Zone through LaughGnosis do so in a way much like people with phobias can unlearn their phobic response. Although the phobic response is learned in a matter of minutes, they carry that phobic response with them every moment of every day. A similar phenomenon can happen with some people through LaughGnosis. Through this process, instead of eliciting a phobic response, a relaxed response can be triggered.

A quick example of such response is as follows: A person who was locked in a closet by their big brother may learn to be claustrophobic in a matter of minutes. In this experience, the subconscious mind automatically links closed in places with the fear associated with the traumatic event, with lifelong effects. Another example would be a veteran who narrowly escaped death when an area 100 yards from him was bombed, and several of his friends were killed. Because coffee was brewing in the kitchen of his barrack at the time of the bombing, he developed a post-traumatic stress disorder (PTSD) that is triggered by coffee.

Just as the association between closed spaces or coffee, and fear of death is learned by some people in a matter of seconds, in the same way the association can be made between laughter and living in a heightened state of awareness in The Zone in one's daily life. This association can be made through LaughGnosis, which we will discuss in more detail in Chapter 23.

Functioning in a heightened state of awareness in The Zone can also be enhanced by practicing a physical skill - like dancing, martial arts or playing music - until the body moves effortlessly and with very fluid movements. These skills can be acquired either through great effort and with anxiety about not being perfect, or through the perfect blend of passion, excitement, determination, and equanimity. When acquired in the second way, they can help us know how to function in The Zone. Once we learn this with one skill, we can practice using that state of mind in our daily life.

Another way to function in a heightened state of awareness in The Zone in our daily life is by practicing the Inconvenient Joke version of mindfulness. Laughing and smiling at The Inconvenient Joke as much as possible can help us become more equanimous. Once we are equanimous, it is often much easier and effective to practice mindfulness - the practice of non-judgmentally paying attention in the present moment in a very focused way.

When practicing mindfulness, we are fully aware of all the details of what we are doing. For example, as we eat, we let go of all other thoughts and bring our full awareness to our food. We notice how good it feels to focus our full attention on the saliva forming in our mouth as we appreciate the fragrances and colors of our food. We take our time to explore all the sensations in our body while we are chewing and swallowing. We bring our awareness to an activity wholeheartedly, no matter how trivial it may seem.

All these ways of achieving a heightened state of awareness in The Zone can help clear away the blockages to our authentic laughter. The authentic laughter can lead us to higher states of awareness and help us live in The Zone.

Smiling: A Way of Preventing "Truth Decay"

This brings us to another ingredient in the FAULTS mnemonic and another way of finding laughter in your daily life: **Smile.**

The "S" for Smile reminds us that – even if it isn't our nature to be uproariously laughing all the time, we can rest in a constant inner smile. This inner smile often shines outwardly to touch and bless whomever we meet.

An authentic and heartfelt smile bubbles over to infect others. It is most potent when it reflects our state of living in The Zone.

We can read all the spiritual books and attend all the spiritual workshops in the world, but until we authentically Smile, all the information we have acquired may just be candy for the ego. If you forget the FAULTS mnemonic, and ignore everything else in this book, at least remember to smile!

The authentic smile is how we know that we are laughing along with God in each moment.

Smiling carries many benefits. Smiling helps prevent tooth decay by exposing the anaerobic bacteria on our teeth to oxygen - which kills them and helps them transition to a more evolved life.

As great minds have said, this world is an illusion that many people take too seriously. When we smile, we help expose this truth, which helps prevent "truth decay."

In each moment, you are either subconsciously hypnotizing others to look at the brighter side of their life and help them join you in The Zone by authentically smiling, or you are encouraging them to look at the darker side by frowning.

As we get in touch with our authentic smile and go through our day smiling from the depths of our heart and soul with everything we do, we may be amazed by the number of people smiling back at us. This will help us smile even more, as we subconsciously hypnotize each other to look at the brighter side of everything with a smiling heart.

Studies have shown that when a person smiles, the physiology of the body changes. The brain decides that we are feeling good and creates more hormones to help us feel even better. As our infectious laughter spreads around the globe, we raise the vibrational frequency of our planet and fulfill our purpose, to do our part to help heal our world.

Laughter

Authentically smiling is an excellent way to provide lubrication for our laughter muscles. But Laughter – "L" of the FAULTS mnemonic – whether at jokes or for no specific reason, helps us open to our authentic laughter at the Inconvenient Joke and at our thoughts.

As a byproduct of laughing, we may experience many health benefits. Dr. Madan Kataria, the originator of "Laughter Yoga," studied the scientific research into the benefits of laughter. This showed that laughter could help many conditions, including heart disease, depression, hypertension, diabetes, arthritis, asthma, allergies, colds, flu, cancer, AIDS, and others[1].

Laughter is good for both mental and physical health. Laughter reduces stress, lowers blood pressure, releases feel-good endorphins, exercises the abdominal and respiratory muscles, and improves cardiac health, among other health conditions. Laughter can also decrease stress hormones, reduce artery inflammation, and increase HDL (the "good" cholesterol).

Researchers in Japan showed that laughter can increase natural killer cell activity. This is important for fighting infections and cancers.

Laughter was also found to lower the level of the stress hormone cortisol which is implicated as a cause of many diseases. It is even thought that laughter causes the release of neurotransmitters that help control pain.

One of the most important findings is the beneficial impact of laughter on inflammation. Inflammation plays a crucial role in many diseases ranging from arthritis to cancer. Inflammation is also a component of many "age-related" chronic diseases that cause disability[2].

A Norwegian study found a significant link between sense of humor and mortality. In an article titled *Laugh Lots, Live Longer* published in Scientific American, researchers found a 48% reduction in death from all causes, with a 73 percent lower risk of death from heart disease and an 83 percent lower risk of death from infection for women. In men, there was a 74% reduction in risk of death from infection[3].

Another study done out of Wayne State University showed that the span of a baseball player's smile can predict the span of his life. Players who didn't smile in their pictures lived an average of 72.9 years whereas players with a beaming smile lived an average of 79.9 years[4]. Also, because smiles are contagious, you are adding joyful years to everyone whose hearts are touched by your smile.

A British study found that one smile can provide the same brain stimulation (as measured by electromagnetic brain scan and heart-rate monitor) as up to 2,000 chocolate bars[5].

Although the health improvements that come from the periodic laughter of the people involved in some of these studies can be helpful, the results may be temporary. The improvement may be reversed if they become re-mesmerized by their Hall of Mirrors.

One of the main reasons for laughing at the Inconvenient Joke is to help us shift into The Zone and into our power. Drunken laughter or laughter at demeaning jokes can take you out of The Zone. Laughing at the Inconvenient Joke, on the other hand, helps enhance a state of equanimity and helps us remain in The Zone.

Thanks

The remaining ingredient in the mnemonic is "**Thanks.**" It is about thanking our Frankenstein Monsters for helping identify our distortions that need cleaning. This "Thanks" should never be forced. But if you feel gratitude toward the challenges in your life for showing you your blockages to Wholeness and for helping you on your Hero's Journey, then, by all means, thank them.

It is helpful to thank our Frankenstein Monsters because they are doing us a service. Everyone we resist is doing us a service by reflecting back to us all the distortions on our lens. **The greater our gratitude for these reflections, the more we align with God's sense of humor, and the easier it is to laugh.**

But the most important person we need to thank is ourselves for being willing to take 100% responsibility for all our Frankenstein Monsters.

When we use Forgiveness, Awareness, Unconditional love, Laughter, Thanks and Smile, our FAULTS can help us laugh at the Powerful Joke, help support our Hero's Journey, and help us find Heaven on Earth.

"God, who sits in Heaven, laughs!"
— Psalm 2:4

Chapter Twenty
Understanding God's Jokes—
The Sherlock Holmes Approach

If your blockages to laughter are deeply hidden in the subconscious mind, putting on your Sherlock Holmes hat can help you find these deeply hidden Jokes of God.

To be on God's side of the Illusory World, we need to tune into His frequency. If God is a comedian, perhaps once we understand His sense of humor, we can step into God's side of The Illusion. Worst case scenario - we'll have some fun with the process.

To understand God's sense of humor, we will use the Sherlock Holmes approach to discovering blockages to laughing at The Joke.

As I mentioned earlier, God's comedy style seems to be irony.

I gave examples of typical Godly humor when we discussed ironies in chapter 16. Now let's take a deeper dive into God's humor using a Shamanistic tool called "The Mitote."

The *Mitote* is a book developed by the Toltec Shamans of ancient Mexico. They used it as a way of "stalking the mind." They described "The Mitote" as "the sound of 1,000 voices in the market place," the babble of the "normal" human mind.

Our job is to incrementally reduce the number of voices in our mind until there is silence. From that silence, we can discover God's hidden Jokes.

The *Mitote* is essentially a tool for examining the distortions on our lens between the Light of God and the Hall of Mirrors. By examining and eliminating these distortions, the *Mitote* can help us live in The Zone and experience many more miracles in our life.

The more we examine and eliminate the distortions, the more we discover that life on Earth may be the greatest Joke in the Universe. If intelligent life is watching us from other planets, we must be their favorite source of entertainment.

The "Mitote Book" is a blank journal. It is a tool to help us examine all the distortions on our lens, and enables us to become aware of the thoughts and beliefs that created each of the distortions in our Hall of Mirrors. By allowing us to see all the reflections that we resist, the Mitote is an excellent way to help us know "Who We Are Not," which gives us a much clearer picture of "Who We Are." Knowing this is the goal of many spiritual teachings. Once we see how we've created each of the distortions and clean them up, we can allow the miracles of God to be reflected back to us.

We begin the process of using the "Mitote book" by first observing our world – the world we are creating in our Hall of Mirrors. We then search our mind deeply to identify each thought that created each aspect of the world that appears to us as Frankenstein Monsters, and write them down. Then, we laugh at the thoughts and their resulting Monsters. As each thought is identified and modified through laughter, we move to other Frankenstein Monsters.

There are four basic steps for using the Mitote to experience more miracles in your life:

1. Identify a person or situation that challenges you and causes a negative emotion.
2. Acknowledge that this negative emotion is the result of a specific distortion on your lens and is being brought to your attention to be healed.
3. Identify the specific thought, belief, agreement, or memory that is showing you the unwanted reflection you are seeing. This may require deep meditation, soul searching, hypnosis, LaughGnosis, and absolute honesty.

4. Decide whether you want to release or modify that thought, belief, agreement or interpretation of a memory considering the negative reflections you are experiencing. Realize that the more these thoughts and beliefs are aligned with the Light of God, the easier it will be for you to live in The Zone.

The "Sybil War" Inside Our Mind

The 1,000 voices in our mind are like the 16 different personalities of Sybil. They are causing chaos in our life from a Sybil War in our mind.

Our job is to use the Mitote exploration to align with the Light of God and make peace with all the warring parts of our personality.

Our other job is to take 100% responsibility for every aspect of this Sybil War inside our mind, even if this results in us facing our worst fears.

Although we inherently have a fear of the Great Abyss or anything that may cause us sadness, we may have an even deeper fear of laughing at God's Jokes.

We are fearful of this laughter because it would shatter our whole illusion of reality and everything we have ever believed. Our identity, our possessions, our history, and everyone and everything we know would completely vanish once we laugh along with God. Yet, it is the most powerful thing we can do. The ability to laugh at God's Jokes is how we know we are taking responsibility for our Sybil War.

Although laughing along with God is the most powerful form of laughter, ordinary laughter is also extremely powerful. This is what Norman Cousins did when he realized his emotions were responsible for his life-threatening disease and theorized that reversing those emotions with laughter could cure it. He didn't allow his fear of taking 100% responsibility for his disease to interfere with his healing.

These are the steps involved in Norman Cousin's self-cure that we can use on ourselves:

1. He noticed the correlation between emotions and his physical condition.
2. He took 100% responsibility for his role in the process.
3. He recognized that since he created the problem, he could correct it.
4. He shifted into his empowered place of choice.
5. Having delved into the Abyss of taking responsibility, he also took the corrective action – laughter.

In Cousins' case, he chose the route of traditional laughter at comedy films. Since traditional laughter can be that beneficial, laughter at God's Jokes must be much more powerful because that laughter helps to liberate us from our Hall of Mirrors.

Here are some more examples of God's Jokes that often go unrecognized:

God's Misunderstood Jokes

A person gets fired from their job and is utterly devastated. When they sit down with their "Mitote" and search their mind for the thoughts that could possibly have created the job loss, they realize that during the weeks before getting fired, they had been despising their job and dreading waking up in the morning to go to work. They wanted to sleep in a few extra hours and then lounge around the house. But when they arrived at work and found out they had been fired, instead of thanking their boss for granting their wish, they went into a deep depression. Once they realize that their thoughts may have created the outer situation, they can ask themselves from the place of choice, "Which did I prefer, sleeping late, or having a job and income?"

Once the person realizes that they created the situation, they are now at a place of choice and can change their thoughts. They can smile at their traumas and dramas and laugh at God's ironies, and manifest new reflections of that elevated state.

Another example would be a person who is feeling unlovable and fears both intimacy and rejection. He wonders why he's never had a long-term, loving relationship and becomes depressed. When he uses "The Mitote," he realizes that instead of feeling depressed, he should be grateful to all his past partners for reflecting his unlovability belief back to him. He also realizes that by not having a long-term relationship with him, his former partners spared him his feared experience of intimacy and rejection. Once he understands how his thoughts may have been responsible for this situation, he can ask, "Is it true that I am unlovable?" He may also ask, "If there is no separate "I," who is it who really gets rejected?"

Instead of feeling totally devastated after being fired or rejected, by using the Mitote, he can understand God's humor. He can see how he may have attracted a particular situation to grant an unconscious wish. The unconscious wish may have been to clear away blockages to living in The Zone. Once these blockages are cleared by laughing at his conditioned thoughts about the situation, this will help him experience more miracles in his life.

Remember that God is doing Her best to provide to us what we subconsciously want or what we subconsciously resist. We interpret some of these responses from God as cruel punishments, but after laughing at them, we see them as ironies and gifts.

Based on the laws of physics, our wishes and prayers are always answered, but in the God version of the Grandest Scheme of answers. When we want abundance or love, God brings situations to our attention that give us the opportunity to let go of any blockages we may be carrying that keep us from discovering the True Abundance and True Love that is a part of the God Essence within us. This Essence is not fleeting and can never be taken away. While these gifts are perceived by us as cruel punishments, God must be trying Her best not to laugh when we get angry at Her for being so cruel. And now that we know all this, instead of getting angry at God, we can laugh along with Her!

Shining the Light on Shadows

Unconscious beliefs implanted from childhood may also be responsible for distorted lenses. A subconscious belief is a belief of which we are not yet aware, but that our mind accepts as true. Such beliefs are often out of alignment with our authentic self. If one of our parents or teachers ever told us that we were ugly, stupid, lazy, or will be a failure in life, that belief can become our truth. Throughout our life, that belief can create our reality - until it is discovered and corrected through the Mitote.

I have been using the Mitote on a regular basis for over 25 years and have found it to be one of my favorite tools. One way I used the Mitote before discovering the power of laughter was in working with extreme feelings I had toward the shadow governments that control world governments. This hatred was a result of my fixed ideas about the way things should be, rather than the way they are. As a result, I felt an intense resistance to doing my taxes, knowing that my hard-earned money was going to fund unnecessary and devastating wars.

My hatred did nothing to change the situation. It only caused me to fall even more out of alignment with the Light of God, causing me even more distortions and more suffering.

After being brutally honest in the use of my Mitote, I recognized that aspects of the "evil shadow government" are the shadow, despicable aspects of myself that I most resist, but which need the most healing. I also realized how they were showing me my mistaken belief that I am a victim of my Hall of Mirrors.

I healed these aspects of myself through equanimity, forgiveness and unconditional love for both myself and for them. I did everything I could to change the objectionable aspects of myself that I saw reflected onto them.

Before this, laughter at this situation seemed difficult. But once I saw the situation from this new perspective, I was able to laugh at it. I felt much more at peace with governments and yet empowered to respond to them from The Zone.

By using the four steps of the Mitote, a person with a health challenge can often identify how their illness may have resulted from a negative emotion. This negative emotion then creates a distortion on their filter which they see in their Hall of Mirrors as the illness. They then identify the specific thought, belief, triggered memory or agreement that is reflected back to them as the health challenge. Once identified, they decide whether they want to release or modify that thought, belief, agreement, or interpretation of a memory in light of the resulting health challenge. During this whole process, they keep in mind that the more any thought, belief, etc. can be aligned with truth, the more likely their condition will change.

Amazed by the Maze

I worked with a woman who had an anaphylactic reaction to kiwi fruit. Even touching a kiwi fruit would cause her to develop a severe rash.

She eventually remembered that she had broken up with her husband while she was eating a kiwi fruit.

With this part of the puzzle uncovered, we used a treatment to neutralize her response to that memory, and from that day forward, she was able to touch and eat kiwi fruits without any problems whatsoever.

The subconscious mind is not very clever. It associates two things without making any logical connection. It saw this painful event and connected it with the kiwi fruit. Using the logic of the subconscious mind, it wanted to do its best to prevent such an event from occurring again. It therefore did everything in its power to stop her from eating kiwi fruit because, according to the subconscious mind, kiwi fruits appeared to be dangerous. Just imagine how many negative correlations your subconscious mind has registered due to unrelated circumstances surrounding traumatic events in your life.

It sounds highly illogical for the subconscious mind to make such associations, but what is most illogical of all is how we allow this illogical, and sometimes dangerous, subconscious mind to run our lives.

A similar pattern can often be identified for a variety of health conditions. When we use the four steps of the Mitote in this way, many health challenges can be changed.

Although we don't know all the contents of the subconscious mind, we can become aware of it by the way we respond to innocuous stimuli like kiwi fruits. Instead of treating the symptoms of these bizarre allergic reactions with medications, it is often best to get out our Sherlock Holmes hat to find and treat its cause.

The mind is a highly intricate maze which continues to amaze. The astonishing thing about our amazing mind is that we make associations virtually every day of our lives, each potentially resulting in similar irrational responses. We can see how easy it is to get lost down the dark rabbit hole of these responses, and how miraculously empowering it is once, (while under the treatment and guidance of one's medical doctor) they are uncovered and miraculously healed.

Questioning God's Ethics

We tend to wonder about God's ethics when we see people who are starving and homeless, people being abused by their partners, or who are being tortured in detention centers.

I feel utmost compassion for those people from the bottom of my heart. But there is a law of Karma which is just as real as the law of gravity. This law is based on Newton's 3rd law: "For every action, there is an equal and opposite reaction." Whatever pattern of energy we produce will ultimately come back to us to equalize the effect. Just like the law of gravity; we can ignore it, but it will eventually come back and bite us.

According to this law, whatever challenges they experience are the result of their past behavior. Their torturous challenge is providing them with the opportunity to work off horrendous past karma. The more they can use those challenges to find equanimity by laughing at their conditioned thoughts, the more karma they will burn and the fewer distortions will remain on their lens. This will help them realign with the Light of

God. Once they realign with This Light, they will be more receptive to Divine Inspiration and will find the miracles that they may not have noticed had they been focused on their suffering.

Another way of looking at those people whose life is an utter Hell is by seeing how they are also showing us what to avoid so we don't wind up like them. Those who are suffering can also help us be grateful for all that we have. They give us the opportunity to share our wealth with them.

For still others, their suffering is essentially like a smoke alarm, alerting them to serious distortions on their lens. The bigger the fire of distortions, the more suffering, and the louder the alarm.

Instead of listening to their alarm and putting out the fire by healing the distortion on their lens, some people resort to drugs, alcohol, food, T.V., the internet or mind-numbing spiritual practices to repress the underlying distortion. They are essentially responding to their fire alarm by turning it off and going back to sleep.

They anesthetize themselves with these vices and feel great - until they wake up to excruciating pain, much more suffering, and a burning desire for even more of those anesthetizing agents. This creates a vicious cycle down into the seemingly bottomless pit of suffering.

In summation, within the non-local reality in which we live, whenever we see something troubling in the world, there is a parallel scenario within ourselves that needs healing.

Laughing Our Way Out of the Illusion

I have been using this Sherlock Holmes approach for over twenty-five years to find the parallel scenarios within myself that needs healing. The more I practice this approach, the less time it takes to find the thoughts that were responsible for challenging situations. When I began using this approach it sometimes took a few days to solve the mystery. I am now finding that as each significant conditioned thought arises, I can often see how it can potentially manifest as people or situations in my life. This realization made it very clear to me about the vital importance of laughing at each significant conditioned thought, as well at the consequences of forgetting.

I found that the deeper I went into uncovering deeply repressed thoughts that attracted the Frankenstein Monsters into my life, the more synchronicities and disguised miracles I discovered, and the more amusing and funnier the game of life became.

Lau Tzu's quote, "As soon as you have made a thought, laugh at it" has morphed into, "As soon as you have made a thought, **find the reason to** laugh at it."

An easy way to laugh at your thoughts and beliefs is by imagining yourself in Heaven, surrounded by angels. Imagine telling God your beliefs that created your Frankenstein Monsters. How long do you imagine it would take Her to burst out laughing?

I am now experiencing Lao Tzu's quote as no longer a rule to follow, but a fun game to play. This process makes challenges seem more like puzzles to solve, and eventually jokes to laugh at. This laughter helps me find many of the hidden miracles and synchronicities that were probably there all along.

Becoming an Alchemist of Our Life

The Mitote is a potent tool. By being brutally honest with our use of the Mitote and doing some intense soul searching, the distortion on our lens can often be identified. On occasion, one may not be able to identify the distortion from this lifetime and may require hypnosis for past life regression.

Once identified, those distortions can be healed in a way that enables us to learn as much as possible from our immense challenges. This empowers us to become the alchemist of our life. This alchemical process transforms the intensity of our suffering into the intensity of our Bliss.

It is important to continue using The Mitote to loosen our blockages to laughter. If instead of this we were to only use positive affirmations and visualizations or incorrectly use the Law of Attraction, we would be falling into the trap of using mind-numbing spiritual practices to repress the underlying distortions that are screaming out to be healed. Ignoring a problem leads to ignor-ance and more suffering.

Much of the chaos we see in the world today may be the result of masses of people improperly using spiritual tools to resist our dark reflections and attract the bright shiny ones. Once we confront our darkness with laughter at the Powerful Joke, that's when we become the alchemists of our life.

Just like Sherlock Holmes did not solve every mystery, neither will you. We are essentially looking at the grand perspective of Universal reality through a pin-hole. We are even blinded by the influence of our own past lives and past karma. We are blinded to how our current challenges are necessary for our spiritual evolution. We also are blinded to how our challenging situation may be beneficial to the totality of All That Is. Perhaps the human race needs to die in order to stop our planet from being destroyed by our treatment of the environment.

Although the Hall of Mirrors and the Frankenstein Monsters are all illusory, we need to continue working on them because they are showing us our blockages to living in The Zone and experiencing all the miracles that can result. If we ignore them, we will become increasingly out of alignment with The Light and may experience much more suffering.

In most cases, it is preferable to learn these lessons on our own terms, when the challenge is small, instead of waiting for life to clobber us over the head with what we have been ignoring. It is also preferable to learn as much as possible through compassion for other people's challenges.

We've had the ability all along to experience inner peace and reclaim our power to make more effective changes in the world. All we needed to do was to use the alchemical power of equanimity, forgiveness, unconditional love, and Powerful Laughter to change anger into authentic power.

Once we clear away any remaining blockages by using FAULTS and The Mitote, we can authentically smile and laugh as an expression of the smile and laughter in our heart.

The Mitote can be the key to identifying and healing the distortions in our lens and may help facilitate miraculous changes in illnesses. It can clean up even the tiniest of distortions on our lens in a very targeted way. Once we enjoy laughing at our Mitote and become the Sherlock Holmes of our life we have done our part toward becoming the masters of our lives. Once this is done, the Light of God will shine directly on our Hall of Mirrors, enabling us to live in The Zone and experience more miracles.

Although FAULTS and The Mitote can be extremely helpful for helping us live in The Zone, the best way to get there is by following the Fifth Noble Truth.

"The human race has only one really
effective weapon, and that is laughter."
— Mark Twain

Chapter Twenty-One
The Fifth Noble Truth

According to Buddha, there are four noble truths:

1. Ordinary life brings about suffering.
2. The origin of suffering and rebirth is craving and aversion.
3. The cessation of suffering and rebirth is attainable.
4. There is a Noble Eightfold Path to the cessation of suffering and rebirth.

These Noble Truths can be very helpful, but also have the potential of making it more difficult to avoid suffering, desires, and rebirth. Too much focus on thoughts about suffering and the elimination of suffering can become a serious effort that creates more suffering, as our serious face is reflected back to us.

Just as our goal is not merely to smile or to experience Bliss, our goal is also not to resist suffering, desires or rebirth.

There is a story about three monks who meet with their teacher for their progress reports. The teacher tells the first monk that because he still has so many cravings and aversions, he will have nine more incarnations. The monk bows and thanks his teacher.

The teacher then tells the second monk that because he doesn't have as many cravings and aversions, he will have four more incarnations. That monk bows and thanks his teacher.

The teacher then walks over to the third monk and tells him that because he has no cravings and aversions, he will have only one more incarnation. That monk says to his teacher, "I have tried so hard to have no cravings and aversions; I thought I would have no more incarnations."

The teacher said, "I made a mistake. You are right. You have tried very hard to have no cravings and aversions in order to have no more incarnations. You now have fifteen more incarnations!"

Trying to eliminate cravings and aversions and preventing suffering and rebirth through the Four Noble Truths may work for some people. For others, it may create more cravings and more resistance that can cause us to be more out of alignment with the Light of God. For those others, my "Fifth Noble Truth" will be especially helpful.

My Fifth Noble Truth is **"Laughter at The Inconvenient Joke is the Best Medicine to end suffering."**

Although the Four Noble Truths and the Noble Eightfold Path are very important, the problem is that most people have an overabundance of cravings and aversions. For those people, The Four Noble Truths and The Noble Eightfold Path may be too subtle to grasp and could create a craving to end craving, and an aversion to rebirth that creates more anxiety throughout their lives.

The Eightfold Noble Path in Buddhism is: Right thought, right speech, right actions, right livelihood, right understanding, right effort, right mindfulness, and right concentration.

Although that all sounds *right*, there is one thing left………laughter.

The attitudes of The Eightfold Path are very noble, however they set up the potential for judgment of ourselves and others. This can be avoided through laughter. This laughter arises as a result of knowing our self as a result of laughing away the illusory self that was based in thought. Once we laugh away all our conditioned thoughts interfering with knowing Who We Really Are, there is no need to try to have right thought, right speech, right actions, right livelihood, right understanding, right effort, right mindfulness, and right concentration.

Once we Know Who We Really Are through any path, we realize that there is no separate me. There is then no need to try to have right thought, right speech, right actions, and so forth; these noble traits happen naturally.

Knowing Who We Are is essentially knowing the version of yourself that has a clear lens. From this space, all actions necessary to follow the Eightfold Path would be expected to arise automatically.

This knowledge of Who We Really Are, which is eternal, also helps eliminate any aversion to rebirth.

The potential problem with the Eightfold Noble Path is that some people have a rebellious part of them that may resist following these rules. Once we know ourselves, meaningful laws become self-evident. Since we see everyone else as a reflection of ourselves, there will be no competition, only cooperation. "Do unto others as you would have them do unto you," will be redundant because why would any sane person want to cheat themselves?

When children are allowed to experience the interconnected reality of Who They Really Are, their core beliefs will be in alignment with their authentic self, and our world will be a much better place.

Instead of leading to this outcome, The Four Noble Truths and the Eightfold Noble Path may have the potential of setting up cravings, aversions and conscious or subconscious rebellion. These tendencies prevent us from progressing on our Hero's Journey and can be responsible for creating more of the suffering which the Four Noble Truths were designed to prevent.

One way to avoid such craving is through my Fifth Noble Truth that "Laughter at the Inconvenient Joke is the Best Medicine to end suffering."

Laughing at the Potential Trap of Buddhism

An aversion to death or rebirth is a reflection of our attachment to our body. Since the body ages and dies, this aversion has the potential to cause suffering – if we forget to laugh at it. But how is rebirth even possible when Who We Really Are, beyond the body, never dies? What is rebirth other than a further re-identification with ourselves as our body? Shouldn't rebirth be a meaningless concept, since Who We Really Are has nothing to do with whether or not we are in one body or another, or in any body at all?

Although one of the intended benefits of the Four Noble Truths is to reduce cravings and aversions, in some people, these efforts can introduce a whole new craving that most people didn't even realize they had. That would be like me telling you there is an Eightfold Path to help you to not think about a mouth-watering chocolate ice cream cake with coconut cream frosting.

Any craving or aversion, as Buddha said, can cause suffering. This includes an aversion to being reborn. Laughterism, on the other hand, can free us from the thoughts that lead to craving and aversion.

"If you become silent after your laughter, one day you will hear God also laughing; you will hear the whole existence laughing with you, even the trees and stones and stars."

— Osho

Chapter Twenty-Two
Laughterism, The Ho-Ho-Holiest Religion

When I was growing up, I questioned a great deal of religious philosophy and dogma. Because of this, I was forced to spend a summer in an intense religious camp, immersed essentially all day in religious dogma during my summer vacation. In some ways, my Vipassana form of torture was the antidote to any remnants of this brainwashing form of torture. The youthful religious indoctrination was agonizing for me because there seemed to be many contradictions that were not thoroughly explained and continued to eat away at my spirit like leeches. It came to the point that I felt so tormented by their brainwashing, that I revolted and went AWOL.

Since that time, I have dabbled in many religions and spiritual philosophies. Although some appealed more than others, I never found any that completely resonated with me, and decided to develop my own. I call this religion Laughterism.

I developed Laughterism despite knowing all too well that one of the problems in the world today is having too many religions that have seemed to result in the creation of more division and potential for Holy wars. I developed Laughterism to help myself and possibly others laugh our way out of the Illusory World and laugh at any thoughts that could evolve into wars.

Laughterism is different from other religions because unlike Judaism, Catholicism, Hinduism, and Buddhism, which have laws or paths to follow, Laughterism has no laws or paths except to enjoy God's Jokes.

Instead of the Four Noble Truths, Laughterism has The Fifth Noble Truth.

Unlike Western societies which believe "I think Therefore I am," Laughterism believes "I Laugh, therefore I Am."

Whereas many Western societies may think their ego-self into existence, Laughterism laughs it right out of existence.

Unlike Judaism and Christianity which have Ten Commandments, Laughterism has only one commandment and one rule. **The one commandment is "Thou Shalt Laugh at The Inconvenient Joke."** From this is conceived the one rule which is "As soon as you have made a thought, laugh at it." From this commandment and this rule, all other behaviors become obvious. Any other commandments and rules are fuel for laughter.

Another difference between Laughterism and other religions is that Laughterism worships Laughter as a way to know God through Her Jokes.

Please note that Laughterism also works as an add on to any other religion you choose. Although you may be expected to keep a more serious external demeanor during some religious services, the internal practice of Laughterism can continue anywhere and everywhere you go.

When we are possessed by laughter at the Inconvenient Joke, we are essentially in a deep meditative state in which thinking stops and a deep sense of peace takes over - like taking a vacation. While it may seem challenging to remain in that state, the more glimpses we have of it, the more normal it becomes. As it becomes more and more normal, it seems easier and easier to stay in that state. New habit patterns benefit from the neuroplasticity of the brain to help us remain in this deeply relaxed state. Instead of trying to rush the process of awakening through laughter at The Powerful Joke, Laughterism focuses on finding The Joke as often as possible.

One way to help this process is by understanding how The Joke may have been forgotten. In our Laughterism mythology, Adam and Eve experienced a deep sense of Peace. This Peace disappeared when they ate from the Tree of Knowledge of Good and Evil - essentially eating the lie that The Illusion is real.

The Laughterism myth of the Adam and Eve story is that in addition to there being a snake in the Garden of Eden, there was also a Laughing Hyena. The Laughing Hyena told Eve about an additional tree, the Tree of Laughter. The Hyena told Eve that eating an apple from the Tree of Laughter is the antidote to eating an apple from the Tree of Knowledge.

As you can guess, in our version of the ten commandments, there is an eleventh commandment. That commandment is, "Thou Shalt Laugh!"

The apple from the Tree of Laughter is always available to you - whether you abide by all Ten Commandments or just the eleventh. Every time you laugh at the Inconvenient Joke, you are taking another bite of the apple from the Tree of Laughter, and one bite closer to waking up laughing.

A meditation that can be used to help in the process of waking up laughing, which is a bit different from long hours of sitting perfectly still in silence during Vipassana meditations, is meditating to the sound of Laughing Hyenas. Look up laughing hyenas or children laughing or laughter yoga videos online and play them as you turn your attention within to connect the outer laughter with your deep inner laughter.

Laughter, The Language of God

Laughterism worships Laughter because it seems to be the language of God.

Although there is holiness in every animal, person and object, the Laughing Hyena is highly regarded because it seems to speak the language of God.

Laughterism agrees with Voltaire, a French Enlightenment writer, who said, "God is a comedian playing to an audience too afraid to laugh."

There was a laughter-related research study led by Lee Berk, an associate professor in the School of Allied Health Professions and an associate research professor of pathology and human anatomy at the Loma Linda University School of Medicine in The United States. The study was conducted on 31 people whose brain wave frequencies were monitored while watching either humorous, spiritual or distressing video clips. The study found that laughter triggers brain waves similar to those related to meditation, and that when watching funny videos, the volunteers' brains had high levels of the same kind of gamma waves that are generated during meditation.

Berk explained that gamma waves are the only frequency found in every part of the brain. He said this means that humor engages the entire brain.

Berk added that, with laughter, "It's as if the brain gets a workout. This allows people to think more clearly and have more integrative thoughts." Berk found that laughter enables people to feel whole or more focused[1].

A study out of Stanford University in the U.S.A. found that this gamma frequency (generated by laughter) is the same frequency as that found in Tibetan monks who had undergone training in meditation for an estimated 10,000 to 50,000 hours, over periods of 15 to 40 years[2].

This Gamma brainwave frequency also synthesizes all the bits of information from various areas of the brain and blends them together in a higher perspective[3].

Gamma brainwave frequency is associated with states of self-awareness, higher levels of insight and information, psychic abilities, and out of body experiences. It is highly active when we are in states of universal love, altruism, and other "higher virtues"[4].

This all sounds like Gamma may be the "God frequency."

It is possible that by keeping Her Jokes hidden, God is encouraging us to find our way to tune into His frequency. We do this by polishing up our special x-ray glasses of Laughter and seeing the world from God's Gamma brain wave frequency. That's when we can find all the Jokes that God plants in our daily lives, Jokes we can only find once we are finely tuned into His frequency.

These studies suggest that it may be possible to achieve the same brainwave frequency with laughter as highly evolved monks do with many years of meditation. The main differences are that we don't need to be confined to a monastery, we don't need to meditate for 40 years, and we can have sex whenever we damn please.

All we need to do is Laugh - and our world becomes our monastery.

Instead of taking a helpless animal to be sacrificed at an altar, Laughterism takes our ego to be altered and sacrificed.

Although you may have groaned at a few of mine, puns may be an additional comedy style of God. It may be His way of encouraging us to tune into His frequency while also showing us how funny our language is.

When I left my ten-day meditation course, I continued having trouble remaining in that meditative state. However, by laughing at The Joke as much as possible, I've been able to take the monastery with me wherever I go.

Laughterism has advantages and disadvantages as a religion.

Seven Advantages

1. It's the simplest *Universal* religion that can be stated in the *Uni-Verse* - "As soon as you have made a thought, laugh at it."
2. Instead of going on guilt trips and worrying about our emotional baggage, we can go on laughter trips and happily lose our emotional baggage.
3. It's the ho-ho-holiest religion.
4. No need to remember any elaborate prayers or mantras. The only mantra is ha, ha, ha, ho, ho, ho, he, he, he, he!
5. Unlike in Judaism where the foreskin is removed, in Laughterism only the ego is removed.
6. Laughterism is a completely non-sexist religion. Everyone has test-tickles.
7. Whereas many religions involve ritualistic meals, Laughterism is greatly enhanced when we are "in-jesting."

Seven Disadvantages

1. If you go ho-ho-ho too hard, you may need to warn Santa before sitting on his lap.
2. You may be restricted to only flying Incontinental Airlines.
3. It's a non-prophet organization.
4. It's the world's most infectious religion.
5. You may be asked for drugs and may be subject to drug testing if you are too happy.
6. If we practice Laughterism too much, we can wind up in the funny farm.
7. Without guilt, fear, and worry - which are integral parts of most religions - you may have trouble convincing others that it is a true religion.

The teaching of our religion is "If you want to live happily ever after, take a bite from the "Tree of Laughter."

Once we are in complete and utter awe of the Cosmic Joke and are diligent in our Laughterism practices, we may see the Joke appearing in more and more places, and it may be difficult to not laugh. Once we know Who We Are, we will find the Joke easier to find wherever we go. It will become more and more evident that the true nature of reality is very different from the version we've believed. Realization of this discrepancy naturally leads to laughter.

After now learning and understanding all the ways to uncover our authentic laughter, it is time to let them go from our conscious mind to our subconscious mind. This is because our subconscious mind controls a majority of our behavior, and because **there is no way to achieve laughter... laughter is the way.**

One way to get this understanding from our conscious mind to our subconscious mind is through LaughGnosis.

> "Out beyond ideas of wrongdoing and rightdoing,
> there is *Bliss beyond measure.*
> *Let's Laugh our way there.*"
> — Inspired by Rumi (with *words in Italic by Mitchell J. Bloom, M.D.*)

Chapter Twenty-Three
LaughGnosis™, the
Ha-Ha-Happiest Path to God

In order to help fulfill my vision of helping mankind laugh its way out of the Illusory World, I developed LaughGnosis. LaughGnosis is a combination of hypnosis and laughter in order to achieve **Gnosis** (God-Realization). I also developed LaughGnosis because I wanted people to be able to attain a similar state of ultimate Bliss beyond words without needing to withstand a near-death experience or agonizing pain from sitting eleven hours per day for ten days without talking or moving. I wanted to develop a fun technique that anyone could enjoy doing. I also wanted to create a process that was grounded in science and transcended religious affiliations. I believed that spirituality need not involve reading hundreds of books or attending spiritual workshops that felt highly inspirational during the process, but had very little carry-over into one's daily life.

I didn't want the process to be a separate activity done at a spiritual retreat, meditation hall, or an ashram. I wanted it to be a way of bringing the ashram experience into our daily life. I wanted a way of bridging our spiritual world with our daily world in a fun and joyful way. I found this could be accomplished with laughter.

I found that, although ordinary laughter alone can be beneficial, there was a significant component of the therapeutic properties of laughter that were missing. Ordinary laughter seemed to be like taking a narcotic for pain.

It often provided short term symptomatic relief but did nothing for the underlying condition.

I wanted to develop a treatment that could be even more effective – one that worked at the subconscious level, the place from which our automatic and habitual thought patterns and behaviors emerge. I wanted to do this in a way that aligns a patient with the Ultimate Healer within each person. For this reason, I developed a way of laughing at God's Jokes, to undo the engrained conditioned thoughts and beliefs responsible for the root causes of some conditions.

I also developed LaughGnosis to help many people, myself included, who have had amazing, mystical, magical, transformational experiences while doing intense meditation or a transformational workshop, yet found themselves returning to their daily life experiencing minimal or no carry-over.

Another reason I developed LaughGnosis is because as Einstein said, "We cannot solve our problems with the same thinking we used when we created them." All these years, I had been focused on treating the physical and emotional components of medical conditions with physical and emotional treatments. My laughter allowed me to let go of my conditioned beliefs about treatment, and sparked the question: what if we can treat conditions at a level beyond the physical and emotional - the place where laughter takes us - through LaughGnosis?

It seemed to me that, although medical interventions are often helpful and necessary, they may not provide the full solution for every patient. Since "We cannot solve our problems with the same thinking we used when we created them," conditions that were created at the physical or emotional levels may require treatments that go beyond those levels to achieve more profound, longer-term results. Trying to fix a patient's condition solely at the physical level for some conditions would be like trying to paint smiles on our Frankenstein Monsters. They might seem to disappear temporarily but may often reappear, or may require ongoing treatment, until addressed at a level beyond the one that created it.

In a world in which every thought creates an aspect of our world, most of our personal problems and worldly problems were created at the level of conditioned thought. One way to help solve these problems is to focus on the level beyond conditioned thought, the level where laughter, meditation, etc. can take us. One way to achieve this can be through LaughGnosis, which can help us access Divine Inspiration.

Another reason I developed LaughGnosis was to bridge the gap between what we know about the nature of reality from our spiritual teachings and Nobel Laureate quantum physicists, versus who we think we are and how we live our lives. I wanted to combine that with my knowledge and experience as a hypnotherapist to improve how we live our lives – lives which are inherently driven by our subconscious beliefs. I developed LaughGnosis to bridge the gap between Who We Really Are, and who we think we are.

I felt as though we had been hypnotized into believing the Illusion of Hell is real. What better way of helping to di-spell this mass hypnotic spell than through the reverse process? LaughGnosis practitioners are not hypnotists.......we are de-hypnotists. We undo the hypnotic spell of the Illusory World.

To be quite honest, this whole philosophical approach to healing came out of my frustration at the minimal changes I saw in myself despite all the inner work I did so diligently, even to the point of risking my life in my near-death experience. Now, after developing and practicing LaughGnosis, I can laugh about that too.

What is LaughGnosis?

LaughGnosis is the combining of laughter with hypnosis to achieve Gnosis. Gnosis is knowing oneself at the deepest level, which, according to some spiritual teachings, is how to know God.

The Gnostic State is an altered state of consciousness in which a person's mind is perfectly focused on one single point, thought, or goal. The gnostic state is used to bypass the "filters" of the conscious mind and is necessary for deep change work.

This is like the state used with hypnosis. In this way, hypnosis may help achieve the "Gnostic State" and can be helpful for profound changes.

Indeed, hypnosis is responsible for some miraculous feats, some of which have helped in the evolution of our world.

If you were to Google "Hypnosis Olympic Gold Medal" you would see a multitude of Gold Medalists and other top athletes who used hypnosis to achieve what others couldn't. In the 1956 Olympics, the Soviet Union topped the medal board with 98. Their secret was that in addition to their regular sports coaches they had 11 additional recruits. These recruits were not sports coaches nor experts in performance-enhancing drugs. They were hypnotists who hypnotized the athletes into becoming super-athletes who almost couldn't help but win.

Other famous people who have used hypnosis include:

Albert Einstein who used trance states to develop his ideas including his theory of relativity.

Thomas Edison used self—hypnosis on a regular basis

Carl Jung and Sigmund Freud developed modern psychiatry as a result of practicing hypnosis.

Mozart composed while hypnotized.

Other people and organizations who have reportedly used hypnosis include Sir Winston Churchill, Jackie Kennedy Onassis, Aldous Huxley The Chicago White Sox, The Swiss Ski Team, Bruce Willis, Tiger Woods, Jimmy Connors, Jack Nicklaus, Sylvester Stallone, Joe Vitale, Julia Roberts, Kevin Costner, and Martha Stewart.

Many people's assumptions are on a collision course with True Reality, the Reality described by Jesus, Nobel Laureates and other geniuses throughout history. By laughing at our false assumptions by using the principles described in my book, we laugh away our blockages to knowing ourselves at the deepest level. By combining the healing power of laughter with the miraculous power of hypnosis, this helps us access our inner Power, our Inner Healer and Divine Inspiration.

LaughGnosis takes hypnosis to a whole new level and is based on the principles presented in this book. The goal is to help the patient joyfully laugh their way out of their world full of traumas and dramas that was created by a belief system based on false conditioned assumptions. Once we do this, we can only imagine what is possible; and what we imagine becomes possible.

LaughGnosis can be a fun way to help access the state used by pro athletes and geniuses who have helped change our world. It can help us laugh our way into the state in which miracles become more possible, a state that can help us create a type of Heaven on Earth.

Why Undergo LaughGnosis?

Hypnosis alone is a highly successful intervention. In 1970, Alfred A. Barrios, Ph.D. conducted a survey of scientific literature to compare recovery rates for various modalities of therapy and found that:

Psychoanalysis can be expected to have a 38% recovery rate after approximately 600 sessions.

Hypnotherapy can be expected to have a 93% recovery rate after an average of 6 sessions.

Ordinary laughter and ordinary hypnosis are highly successful interventions when done alone. When used in conjunction with the consciousness and philosophy described in this book, the results can be even better. When used by a certified LaughGnosis practitioner, the results may be even better still. Unfortunately, as of the writing of this book, there aren't many LaughGnosis practitioners, but as the idea catches on, we hope to train many more. Visit HoHoHoly.com for more information about receiving training or treatment.

LaughGnosis, when combined with medical approaches under the supervision of your doctor, can often effectively treat a problem at the deepest root psycho-emotional-spiritual level. When this occurs, not only is the presenting problem effectively corrected on a long-term basis, other problems are corrected as well. Also, the patient will feel much more peaceful, integrated and Whole as they appreciate their condition as a part of their Hero's Journey. This will result in a sense of peace, and greater ability to function from within The Zone.

For example, a patient presents with cancer pain. Through some discussion or through hypnosis it becomes clear they experienced major challenges shortly preceding their diagnosis. They soon realize that their cancer pain is the call to adventure on their Hero's Journey discussed in chapter 14. After exploring the lessons behind their cancer on the subconscious level (while continuing to undergo any necessary medical treatments), not only may the cancer pain resolve, but they may feel more peaceful and Whole moving forward.

The subconscious mind is the level at which our behavior and physiological responses to challenges can predispose us to disease. Until the core responses are reframed and changed at this level, dramatic improvement may be less likely.

Going through a major disease can be a very challenging Hero's Journey that nevertheless becomes worth the pain once we use that challenge to transform, heal and laugh at any possible predisposing thoughts.

People can spend thousands of dollars over many lifetimes on their spiritual development. Even if they totally understood all these teachings, it may have minimal effect on the person's behavior, because most teachings tend to work on the conscious level.

Within a few sessions of LaughGnosis, this can be changed, not only at the conscious level but also at the subconscious level, where it may have an impact for lifetimes and generations to come. It can impact the way we bring up our children and how those children bring up their children. It can also have a significant impact on everyone around us, and those around them, etc.

Practicing LaughGnosis on others as a LaughGnosis practitioner can have an even more profound impact on the practitioner because what we teach, we learn.

More benefits of LaughGnosis

1. Can address the root cause of many conditions.
2. Can provide longer lasting, safer and more effective results – when combined with medical treatment.
3. Can save many years of therapy, spiritual education, and workshops.

4. Helps us access our Inner Healer.
5. Quickly helps the patient and the practitioner know Who They Really Are at deeper levels.
6. Helps the patient and the practitioner feel unconditional love, which is free of guilt and fear.
7. Can improve health and quality of life.
8. Can help the patient live a longer and happier life.
9. Promotes a deep sense of peace that can never be taken away from you, regardless of the circumstances.
10. It's essentially a way of making your own natural, FREE drugs for the rest of your life.

Does the Patient Need a Spiritual or Religious Background?

LaughGnosis was developed so that anyone can benefit regardless of their degree of spiritual background or religious affiliation. It is non-denominational and nonsectarian. It can be used whether the person is Christian, Buddhist, Hindu, Atheist, or any other creed or religion.

What is Hypnosis?

Hypnosis is not like what you see in the movies. It is a natural state of selective, focused attention that is entirely natural and normal. Our ability to enter this unique state of consciousness opens the door to countless possibilities for healing, self-exploration and profound change. Hypnosis has been recognized for thousands of years and used for many purposes.

When we enter into hypnosis, we can use our thoughts, talents, and experiences in ways not usually available to us. We can develop innate abilities to make desired changes in our thoughts, feelings, and behaviors. Hypnosis allows us to regain control of "automatic" behaviors that we could not ordinarily consciously change.

Hypnosis has been successfully used in the treatment of pain, depression, anxiety, stress, habit disorders, and many other psychological and medical problems.

Ten Myths About Hypnosis

Myth #1: The Hypnotist will be able to control my mind.

Fact: No one can control your mind unless you let them. Hypnosis is a way to regain more powerful control of your mind in a way that is safe and effective. If you hear a suggestion that you don't agree with or don't understand, your subconscious mind will automatically reject it, or just laugh at it.

Myth #2: I will be made to perform embarrassing acts, such as bark like a dog, or walk like a duck.

Fact: This assumption is based on Stage Hypnotism and Hollywood fiction. The truth is, stage hypnotists screen their volunteers to select those who are cooperative, with possible exhibitionist tendencies, as well as responsive to hypnosis. These selected subjects allow themselves to participate in acting out silly suggestions. Stage acts have created a myth about hypnosis that discourages people from seeking legitimate hypnosis. Hypnosis is a process of self-improvement, not entertainment, although you may find during your LaughGnosis session that you are the most entertaining actor of all!

Myth #3: Hypnosis comes from "Black Magic" or is "Supernatural."

Fact: Hypnosis is a natural state that has been studied scientifically and validated. Hypnotists are not psychics or palm readers with "special powers." Hypnosis is based on many years of clinical research by famous psychologists such as Dr. Sigmund Freud, Dr. Carl Jung, and Dr. Milton Erikson.

Myth #4: Hypnosis is a "Miracle Cure."

Fact: While Hypnosis is a relatively quick method of making natural and permanent changes, there is no guarantee of a one-time miracle cure. Everyone makes progress at their own rate. The more you incorporate the principles of this book, the faster your progress will be.

Myth #5: I have never been in Hypnosis before.

Fact: Everyone naturally enters a state of hypnosis at least twice every day: just before falling asleep at night, and upon awaking every morning, before getting out of bed. Most people easily enter "Environmental Hypnosis" states while watching TV, driving on the highway, or reading a good book.

Myth #6: Hypnosis is a great tool to get someone to "confess."

Fact: Hypnosis sessions are kept private and confidential. It cannot force anyone to "tell the truth" or to confess.

Myth #7: Self-Hypnosis is safer, better, or more effective than going to a trained professional.

Fact: Self-Hypnosis can be detrimental when not done by a trained professional. A negative attitude or belief about oneself can be reinforced regardless of suggestions given and can cause more problems in the long run.

Myth #8: I can't be hypnotized because my mind is too strong.

Fact: The opposite is most often the case. A person with a strong mind can use this strength to allow the hypnosis to work more effectively and will get more out of each session. The stronger their will to change, the more effective the session will be when properly aligned with their higher purpose and the Will of God (which will be discussed before the session).

Myth #9: When hypnotized, I will lose all sense of my surroundings, and will have no memory of the session.

Fact: Hypnosis is not an unconscious state of sleep. In fact, most people report having a heightened sense of awareness, concentration, and focus. Hypnosis can give you a much higher perspective of reality that may be considered one step closer to God's perspective. Laughter can help this process.

Myth #10: Hypnosis is Dangerous. If I become Hypnotized, I may not be able to "*snap out of it.*"

Fact: Hypnosis is very safe and is, in fact, a state of hyper-awareness. Any time there is an emergency, a person would naturally be able to come out of hypnosis by merely opening their eyes and stretching or speaking.

The whole purpose of LaughGnosis is to help you *snap out of the Grand "It"* which is the "Illusory World" we call our reality.

Christian Views of Hypnosis

The Roman Catholic Church has issued a statement approving the use of hypnosis. In 1847, a decree from the Sacred Congregation of The Holy Office stated, "Having removed all misconceptions, foretelling of the future, explicit or implicit invocation of the devil, the use of hypnosis is indeed merely an act of making use of physical media (that are otherwise licit) and hence it is not morally forbidden, provided it does not tend toward an illicit end or toward anything depraved."

The late Pope Pius also gave his approval of hypnosis. He stated that the use of hypnosis by health care professionals for diagnosis and treatment is permitted. In 1956, in an address from the Vatican on hypnosis in childbirth, the Pope gave these guidelines:

1. Hypnotism is a serious matter, and not something to be dabbled in.
2. In its scientific use, the precautions dictated by both science and morality are to be used.
3. Under the aspect of anesthesia, it is governed by the same principles as other forms of anesthesia.

This is to say that the rules of good medical practice apply to the use of hypnosis.

Some in the Christian Church oppose hypnosis because they say it has been used by the occult. Yet prayer, which has also been used for occultist purposes, is promoted.

The fact is, everything can be used for good or evil. Some lawyers, chiropractors and physicians can work wonders, while others cause much harm. Doesn't it make the most sense to choose the most ethical doctors and therapists to use the most powerful tools in the most constructive ways to achieve the most exceptional results?

Others in the Christian Church oppose hypnosis because they believe it is a form of mind control. Yes, it is true that it is a form of mind control, but one that returns powerful control back to the person undergoing hypnosis. Without hypnosis, our unconscious habits control us. Hypnosis helps the patient to regain control of prior limitations and bodily conditions that were unconsciously acquired over their lifetime, to help regain control of their lives.

Hypnosis is very safe. People will not do or say anything in trance that they would not normally do or say in their normal waking state. This can be seen in the following examples:

The Safety of Hypnosis

There is a story about Milton Erickson telling his secretary that he wanted to rest, so if anyone called, she was to tell them he was out of the office. She agreed to do this. Several days later Dr. Erickson put his secretary into a hypnotic state. When he made the same request, she responded that she could not fulfill it. When asked "Why," she responded, "Because it would be a lie." The secretary had stronger morals under hypnosis than in her normal waking state.

I have a friend who is an excellent hypnotic subject. Because of this, many hypnotists have chosen her for their demonstrations. One day she did a demo on being a human bridge, in which she was lying face up between two chairs, while someone stood on her abdomen, something she would not have normally been able to do. This demonstration was highly successful. Before bringing her out of trance, however, she was given the suggestion that upon awakening, she would cluck like a chicken. Because this was something she would not do in her waking state, she did not come out of trance. It wasn't until the hypnotist reversed this suggestion that she was able to pop right out of trance. Even though she cooperated with the most difficult suggestions, she did not cooperate with the easiest, because clucking like a chicken was a suggestion she subconsciously rejected.

Along with being approved by the Pope and The Roman Catholic Church, hypnosis has been scientifically validated[1]. Used properly, it can be beneficial to your emotional, physical, and spiritual well-being. When combined with laughter in the form of LaughGnosis, it can be a powerful way of accessing the God Essence, the Ultimate Healer within us.

"In the end, everything is a gag. Life is funny. God is funny. You're funny. The events of this world are funny. Joy is funny, love is funny, and as some have discovered after intense troubles, even suffering can be funny when you have the benefit of hindsight."
— Sharon Janis, Spirituality For Dummies

Chapter Twenty-Four
Laughing Our Way to Heaven

In the end, the Joke is on me. I spent much of my life trying to attain the American Dream, helping my patients' pain, and resisting the Great Abyss which unknowingly was binding my chains more and more tightly to the Illusion of Hell. By skedaddling to the other side of the world to escape a presidential administration I found unbearable, the Great Abyss that I tried to escape became much more inescapable and abysmal. It was just another one of God's Inconvenient Jokes once I understood His sense of humor.

In many ways, I felt like Dr. Victor Frankenstein. I devoted my whole life to running and resisting and thereby inadvertently creating even more Frankenstein Monsters. Now, after seeing their seemingly destructive character, I am spending the rest of my life trying to undo my creations.

Victor Frankenstein was a very arrogant and ego-driven doctor. He had a desire to create life, and therefore to be like God.

Although everyone was afraid of Frankenstein's Monster, the Monster's true nature was not destructive at all. It was only when he felt threatened or when he judged himself as ugly that he became violent. Indeed, the Monster loved his creator, Victor.

Perhaps our Frankenstein Monsters are also misunderstood. They only become violent and destructive when we misunderstand their real purpose - of showing us what's blocking us from experiencing a much better world than we've imagined possible.

Instead of learning from these Monsters while they are still cute and small, we misunderstand them. Thus, the Monsters need to become scarier, until they get our attention. Hopefully we will understand God's sense of humor and learn from our Monsters before it's too late.

Unlike Dr. Victor Frankenstein, who only created one Monster, I'd created heaps of Frankenstein Monsters, all over the globe – within my mind.

In many ways, I was even worse than Dr. Frankenstein. Unlike Victor Frankenstein who only desired to be like God, I wanted to create a world better than God's. In my pursuit of the American Dream, I resisted God's lessons. But whenever we try to be like Victor and be like God, can we ever be a true........*Victor*?

Instead of realizing this, I continued sitting in front of my mirrors thinking that one day, if I tried hard enough and had enough luck, if I read enough spiritual books and attended enough spiritual workshops, I would be able to create a better world than the one God intended. I whole-heartedly believed the world I created would take advantage of all the technological advances, despite how much they pollute and destroy the planet and try to over-ride the world God intended. This put me more out of alignment with the Light of God and lo and behold, scarier Monsters appeared, driving me into a Greater Abyss. I was essentially shouting at God, "My will, not Thy Will." To this God was essentially replying, "We'll see."

Waking Up from The American Nightmare

With 20/20 hindsight, I see that I entered the Hall of Mirrors and became very entranced by my desire to live the American Dream. I wanted to create a Dream that would bring me more Bliss than the one God had intended.

This resulted in The American Nightmare, consisting of horrifying Monsters that caused me great fear. I didn't know how to escape. Since everyone else seemed to be seeing similar Monsters, I believed seeing

Monsters is normal. I had not an iota of a clue that a Monster-free world was possible. And to top this all off, I didn't even realize I was mesmerized by my Hall of Mirrors.

During most of my life, I was secretly wishing that I had everything the Global Elite had, including all the social conditioning that would have justified this behavior, believing that I would be just as happy as them. I failed to realize that many of them are more miserable than I ever was, hated by millions of people around the world, needing 24/7 bodyguards, and creating horrifying karma of Hell that may take their soul an eternity to clear.

As another part of my vision of the American Dream, I idolized people like Marilyn Monroe, Michael Jackson and Elvis Presley, whose Frankenstein Monsters were terribly misunderstood.

I and those I idolized were trying to create Hall of Mirrors that was infinitely better than the one God intended, secretly believing that this would make us the happiest. In the process of trying to create this mega Shangri-La, we ignored the Light of God which, if allowed to shine on our Hall of Mirrors, would be infinitely better than any Shangri-La we could imagine. In this process, we were entirely out of alignment with the Light and suffered the consequences.

I lived a life of "Disempowered Resistance" to what is. I spent much of my life trying to create better-looking reflections, only to find even scarier Monsters. If instead, I would have laughed at the Inconvenient Joke and at my thoughts, I could have changed "Disempowered Resistance" into "This-empowered Laughter."

I entered my Hall of Mirrors in search of the American Dream but became so en-tranced by its en-trance, I lost its exit.

Marilyn Monroe, Michael Jackson, and Elvis Presley were each a great teacher. They died sad deaths, despite attaining the American Dream. I believed that if I kept working hard enough, then I too would achieve the American Dream and would live happily ever after. After all, isn't this the promise implied in the American Dream fairy tales? Although I previously never questioned these fairy tale beliefs, they subconsciously ruled my life.

Global Chaos: The Punchline with a Mighty Punch

I regret to admit that the reason I despised the Global Elite so much was that I had initially perceived them as also wanting to create a better world at the expense of others. They were my gruesome shadow side I so much wished to hide - so I projected my anger onto them for many years. These poster children for the great American Dream seemed more like poster children for the great American Shadows who were responsible for the great American Nightmare.

They are showing us that we may wish to reconsider our collective desire to create a better world than God intended at the expense of all else.

Another reason I despised the Global Elite so much was that I had a sense of feeling enslaved, oppressed, abused, overburdened and overworked. I felt as if I was being milked by them and paying high taxes to support their corrupt and lavish lifestyles. It is very tempting to secretly wish them negative karma. But the degree to which we have these deeply hidden desires will be reflected back to us in our karma in the same intensity as our wishes.

I continued to share in a consensus belief in lack and limitation. This belief is the one driving the fundamental law of economics – the law of supply and demand. The belief in lack and limitation results in a perceived lack of supply. This can result in the belief that we can only earn a living at the expense of someone else in this perceived dog-eat-dog world.

This belief in lack and limitation can be reflected back as design structures of planned obsolescence in which a product or service has an artificially limited useful life. They become obsolete, unfashionable, or no longer functional after a certain period of time. This belief helps to generate long-term sales.

This is the reason a car, a lightbulb, or an energy source that can last very long has never made it to market. It is just not profitable long-term and is ignored.

The Global Elite and the whole economic system were doing their jobs perfectly, creating a punchline with a mighty punch. On a personal level, they were perfectly reflecting back to me my belief in lack and limitation. They were also reflecting back to me a distorted idea that in order to make a nice living, one needs to be corrupt. Once I was completely honest with myself, I noticed how I was taking advantage of others in a very attenuated but similar way as the Global Elite, or that I might have done so, given the opportunity. Many years ago, I was providing highly paid services that helped to alleviate symptoms but were not effective at treating the root causes of conditions, even though I knew there was an alternative that could be safer, more effective and longer lasting. While exploring my shadows, I saw my underlying fear that if I did provide the most effective services to restore their health completely, I would earn less, or even put myself out of business.

This brought up a main concern. Once we can experience miracles, this will be inconvenient to those who profit from people who are suffering.

Those very dangerous thoughts of putting myself and others out of business went under the radar. These unlaughed at thoughts triggered an unrecognized fear that mysteriously delayed the release of this book until that fear was finally recognized. This delay materialized as finding reasons to make numerous adjustments to the text and front cover of the book and finding the wrong cover designers. I was subconsciously concerned about being essentially crucified in some way for threatening the livelihoods of those in the most powerful positions. Until I recognized that thought and laughed at it, I planned to protect myself by adding a note to some of those powerful people that went something like this:

I was going to invite some powerful people to take a few moments to notice all the times they attacked or took advantage of others. I wanted them to fully observe what that truly accomplished, and how that will make them feel when they look back at their actions on their death-bed. I was also going to invite them to take a few moments to imagine what it would feel like to let go of all beliefs in separation, and all other conditioned lies as determined by Nobel Laureates and the wisest people who ever lived. I wondered:

- If their conditioned behavior, which was on a collision course with reality, was getting them what they wanted; or whether they would find that their happiness was always right around the corner, never to be found.

- How long it would take them to discover for themselves that what they seem to be doing to others is what they are, at some level, doing to themselves within this interconnected reality in which we live.

- How they would feel if they woke up and found our roles reversed in a future lifetime.

- If their subconscious mind would create a continuing Illusion of Hell until they worked off their karma.

- If they were ready to let go of their conditioned thoughts and behavior to discover the Heaven that may be possible should they decide to explore *__Divine Laughter.__*

- How long would it take them to fully understand that in order to be Truly happy within our interconnected reality, we need to embrace our interconnectedness by loving each other as ourselves.

Delivering the Knockout Punchline

After writing that oh-so-benevolent message to my Frankenstein Monsters, I felt as though waves of laughter were tickling every cell of my body until I just about felt like rolling on the floor as the full impact of the Joke finally struck me at my core. The hypocrisy of inviting "others" to see the fallacy in their illusion of "others" seemed utterly hilarious, especially in light of everything I had written in this book. I had forgotten to take my own medicine and suffered a terrible dis-ease: a fear of "other" people. I had fallen into Hell, forgetting that Nobel Prize laureate Jean-Paul Sartre said that "Hell is other people."

Finding happiness in a world of "other" may be utterly impossible. Seeing the perfectly interconnected parts of ourselves as "other" is the cause of our uttermost suffering and is utterly hilarious. Some of the wisest people who ever lived told us of our Interconnectedness. To them, the illusion of "other" would sound hilarious. Once we embrace our Interconnectedness by laughing at our illusion of "others," we laugh our way Home to Heaven on Earth.

Instead of remembering to laugh at the illusion of "other," that benevolent message to my Frankenstein Monsters was trying to protect "other people" from "other people." I was essentially double-dipping into the Hell created by the illusion of "other people."

The illusion of "other people" who are separate from me was the unlaughed at Joke that kept me in Hell. I had forgotten that the idea of "utter people" is "utterly" hilarious. This hilarious idea was responsible for all the Hellish aspects of my world.

But once we fully embrace the truth, that we live in a non-local reality in which everything is interconnected and laugh at the utterly hilarious illusion of "other people," we deliver the Knockout Punchline to our illusory world and laugh our way from Hell to Heaven.

That Knockout Punchline knocked some sense into my head and enabled me to see the world more clearly. Instead of saying, "Forgive them, Father, for they know not what they do," I began saying, "Thank You, Father, for 'they' know exactly what 'they' do." All my Frankenstein Monsters were doing "their" best to show "me" the consequences of forgetting to laugh at the illusion of "other people." "They" were helping "me" in "my" evolution from Hell to Heaven. I trust that as I continue to laugh, this process will continue to enable karma to be burned in a gentle and joyful way for the highest good of all my perceived fragments.

When we transition from asking God to forgive "them" to thanking God for sending us such a hilarious joke, we are essentially laughing in the faces of our Frankenstein Monsters. This laughter is like throwing water on the Wicked Witch of the West and watching the illusion of "other" Frankenstein Monsters melting away before our very eyes.

A Course in Miracles says, "Into eternity, where all is one, there crept a tiny, mad idea, at which the Son of God remembered not to laugh." In our forgetting to laugh, we took this "tiny mad idea" seriously, and it became our reality. Once we deliver this Knockout Punchline by laughing at our illusion of separation, the game of Hell is over, and we are truly free and liberated people. We are liberated from our conditioned illusion and from believing that it could ever be possible to be the victim of "other people."

The good news is that we are gifted with the English language in which The Knockout Punchline is embedded in practically every sentence. Almost every sentence has a noun or pronoun. These nouns or pronouns and all the Frankenstein Monsters they create, provide a constant source of laughter at our old conditioned illusion of "others." Every time we laugh at a noun or pronoun, or any Frankenstein Monster they create, we feel better and better, and it gets easier and easier to laugh our way out of the illusory world of separation and into living in a Heaven on Earth.

As we wake up laughing to the surprise of the discovery of the interconnected nature of our reality, and the realization that life cannot be against us because we are life itself, we deliver the Knockout Punchline of our illusory world. As we continue delivering the Knockout Punchline, we box our way out of our isolated box of separation and become the heavyweight champions of our illusory world.

Bursting the Spiritual Bubble

For many years, I fell into a trap. I did a great deal of spiritual exploration with a variety of different teachings, believing I could become spiritual and achieve enlightenment, or some such nonsense. It wasn't until many years later that I admitted to myself that this was yet another sneaky way for my ego to again assert, "My will, not Thy Will." It resulted from an aversion to suffering and a craving for a better life.

The same spiritual practices that were supposedly designed to help my spiritual growth were the very practices that hampered it most. Those practices were my spiritual way of avoiding the Great Abyss that was necessary for my progression on my Hero's Journey.

My spiritual practices caused me to live in a spiritual bubble. My spiritual practices were my "aversion" to the truth, instead of "a version" of my truth. It was my aversion to a version of the truth I resisted because it would force me to face my Abyss by forcing me to face my delusory fears. Instead of laughing away those fears, I chose a version of the truth I experienced through spiritual filters. This provided me with a delusional bubble that would burst with the first unexpected challenge.

My subsequent experiences helped me realize that my spiritual consumption was delicious super-food for my super-ego, but kept me locked up in my head, boarded up in my thoughts, thinking I was oh so spiritual.

I finally realized as a result of my near-death related experiences that the world beyond The Illusion cannot be understood through the filters of thought. It needs to be experienced from a place beyond the mind. Any thoughts that were stimulated by books and workshops that caused me to see the world through spiritual filters created more distance to the exit from the Illusory World.

I realized that I had categorized certain activities as spiritual and others as non-spiritual. But when I let go of such judgment and categorization through laughter, I experienced the God essence within everything. I realized that I need not go to an Ashram to Awaken. The world does an excellent job of giving guidance and showing me my blockages to Awakening.

I realized that the way to experience a place beyond the mind and beyond the Illusory World is by seeing the truth as it really is beyond my thoughts. I found laughing at my thoughts to be a fun way of shifting past them.

One of my most important discoveries was not to try to escape the Illusory World because that kind of craving-based effort would make the process much more difficult. Instead, I found it helpful to laugh at all my thoughts about ever escaping.

Although ordinary laughter is helpful, laughing at The Inconvenient Joke is the nuclear bomb for the destruction of the Illusory World. **Asking the mind to sort this out through spiritual teachings is like asking members of Congress to tell the truth in order to put themselves out of a job.**

The mind has a vested interest in creating dramas to keep itself in power. The best way to break out of its spell is spelled l-a-u-g-h-t-e-r.

Some spiritual books and workshops can be very beneficial, but many of them work at the level of the mind. The mind, because it doesn't want to put itself out of business, has many tricks up its sleeve. **Therefore, the mind cannot be transcended at the level of the mind.** It can best be transcended by working at a level beyond the mind, in line with Einstein's observation that, "We can't solve problems by using the same kind of thinking we used when we created them."

Laughter is a magical tool that gets us outside the mind, beyond the level at which the problem was created. Laughing at the Inconvenient Joke allows us to laugh at the mind. Since it silently silences the mind, there is no resistance.

Global Evolution through Laughter

One way to imagine how global evolution can take place is through quantum entanglement. Quantum entanglement is a physical phenomenon that occurs when pairs or groups of particles interact in ways such that the quantum state of each particle cannot be described independently. This explains how two particles can instantly communicate, regardless of the distance between them.

Every time we laugh at the Inconvenient Joke with another person, our souls may be joining beyond the mind, in a very powerful "field." This may result in quantum entanglement and rewiring of the neural networks of our brains in a way that helps both of us wake up laughing. The more we do this, and the more people who share our laughter, the more neural rewiring can take place. At that point, neuroplasticity can take place, and the rewiring of these neural networks can become more solidified.

Because of the infectious nature of laughter, this positive kind of entanglement may be enhanced. As this spread continues, laughter can dissolve the conditioned thoughts, judgments and beliefs that appear to separate us. As this continues, the old conditioned thoughts of the ego that seemed to divide us can slowly melt away and allow humanity to melt away into all of existence.

We can then meet each other in that magical "field" Rumi described, "out beyond ideas of wrong-doing and right-doing," where we share the antidote from the Tree of Laughter. This growing shift could allow humanity to go well beyond our old way of thinking and begin truly solving our problems with a different way of thinking than the way that created them.

By coming together in that field of laughter, we can interconnect at the deepest level of our soul, in that field that exists well beyond our usual thoughts of intimacy. As we continue to join our souls together in that deepest and most intimate field of our collective psyche and continue laughing at the Inconvenient Joke, we can implant The Joke into those around us, impregnating them with the seeds of laughter necessary for them to also wake up laughing. This can lead to the birth of a new world of Heaven on Earth, beyond our wildest conception.

According to A Course in Miracles, we conceived of and bought into the Illusory World by remembering not to laugh. Let's reverse this process by remembering to laugh.

It is up to each of us to infect everyone we meet with this wonderful "chi" energy of laughter. This is easy to do because the energy of laughter is contagious. It encourages others to be copy cats, which makes the energy of laughter so "cat-chi."

Going Forward

As a result of living as the interconnected beings we inherently are, I envision a future in which we all set aside our perceived differences and work together for the greater good of everyone and everything in existence. Some industries will become obsolete while others would expand and flourish, and new ones will be born. Restructuring and retraining for businesses would be funded through "Karma Dollars" – money collected from penalties imposed on illegal businesses. The new currency could be the "Love" instead of the dollar. Instead of competition and greed, we would all want to "spread the Love," so that everyone could thrive. The economy could be measured in GDL: "Gross Domestic Love."

Instead of our two political parties coming together and dividing a nation, they could come together to laugh at all the perceived problems we created by believing division is possible.

Instead of something being considered expensive, it could be considered deserving of a lot of love. Instead of spending a lot of money, people could see it as giving a lot of gratitude with "Love." Instead of costing an arm and a leg, purchases would be deserving of your heart and soul. Instead of having an economy based on lack and limitation led by economists, we could live in a world of cooperation and Love, resulting in global prosperity on every level and led by enlightened masters.

We need to face the fact that some people, industries and political organizations will become overwhelmingly fearful about going forward in this manner. Whether the "others" represent other people, animals, or our planet Earth, they would be afraid that if they no longer exploited "others," they would go out of business. By failing to laugh at the fearful thoughts that will inevitably arise during this transitional period, they would likely suffer emotional trauma.

I believe they will finally realize that their conditioned thoughts are on a collision course with the true nature of our Interconnected reality. They will eventually understand that they will inevitably face the consequences of the physical law of karma and suffer the Hell of the illusion of "other people," Once they do, they will know they have at least one rational choice. That choice, among other choices, will be to use the tools in this book to laugh at their conditioned Hellish thoughts.

The more they laugh at their conditioned thoughts, the more likely they will be receptive to Divine Intuition which will guide them to a career that will be the best for all concerned. Because there are no separate entities, "the best for all concerned" benefits Them, the "Them" that is Interconnected with All That Is. Once they successfully make this heroic transition, the world will be transformed into a type of Heaven on Earth.

Does this sound like a lofty vision?

Maybe, but it is a vision based on solid facts. Once we see "ourself" as one cell within an infinite being, we will no longer come together as communities needing some sort of barter system. We will naturally come together out of an expression of loving our interconnection. We will work in a similar way as a heart cell works to pump blood to nourish the whole body and harmoniously receive nourishment from the other cells of the body without giving anything a second thought.

Once everyone on the planet finally embodies our interconnected nature, all the terrorists, corrupt business and world leaders will realize the consequences of their actions. They will laugh at their antiquated ways of seeing their world that never seemed to give them what they Really wanted – a feeling of Global Love, Unity, and Bliss that is so overwhelming, it makes you want to cry.

Can you imagine what the world would look and feel like waking up in the morning and going through your day - today.....one month..... three months.....six months.....one year.....and five years from now once everyone is guided by Divine Inspiration? Can you imagine what it would sound like as you listen to the news and hear how our global leaders and politicians have joined forces with local groups to help each other achieve our highest potential in our relationships with our family, our friends and our community in a way that is mutually loving and nurturing? As a result of this global shift, can you imagine what advances can be made in technology, and what it would look like and feel like to continue this process as long as necessary until you are ready to transcend the world of time and space to enter other Heavenly dimensions?

I invite you to spend some time to let go of your conditioned thoughts about what is possible, and to consider what we can experience once we explore the Power of Divine Laughter and create a world guided by Divine Inspiration.

Yes, this vision may seem lofty. But once we Laugh away our perceived separation, embody our true interconnected reality, open ourselves up to Divine Inspiration, and put this into practice in our world, this lofty vision may become our blissful reality.

Saying Goodbye to The Illusory World

Infectious laughter at the Inconvenient Joke on a global scale is one way of accomplishing this lofty goal. It is the bottom card that, once pulled, will bring down the house of cards of the Illusory World.

Laughter is the rainbow that bridges the world of the Illusory World with this magical world that appears to be over the rainbow. I invite you to help bridge those two worlds by laughing as much as possible at The Inconvenient Joke.

In the vision I've had since experiencing, researching, and contemplating my epiphanies and experiences, I see laughter at our thoughts and the Inconvenient Joke as our key to Heaven before we die. We can use it to unlock a world full of miracles. Laughter at each thought is our skeleton key to the exit door of the Illusory World.

Laughter is also our skeleton key to open the graveyard so we may return our Frankenstein Monsters to where they belong. It is also our skeleton key to Heaven before we become a skeleton.

Therefore, our story has a happy ending. The best ending for any Frankenstein storyline is one that ends with a cemetery plot.

The good news is, there will never be another Frankenstein Monster. Frankenstein can never have children because.......his nuts (and bolts) are in his neck!

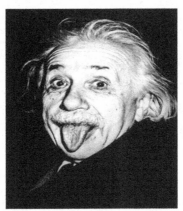

Image of Albert Einstein taken by
United Press photographer Arthur Sasse in 1951.

Now our job is to see nouns and pronouns and our remaining Frankenstein Monsters as reminders to laugh at the frank teachings of EINSTEIN. When we see our world that is filtered through our conditioned thoughts juxtaposed onto the frank EINSTEIN teachings, this will cause us to laugh at our FrankEINSTEIN Monsters. Whenever we see another noun or pronoun or Frankenstein Monster, it can as serve a reminder to remember these frank teachings of Einstein:

"Reality is merely an illusion, albeit a very persistent one."

"Our separation of each other is an optical illusion of consciousness." (we live in a non-dualistic illusion)

"Time and space are modes by which we think and not conditions in which we live."

"I want to know God's thoughts; all the rest are just details."

"We cannot solve our problems with the same thinking we used when we created them."

"Insanity is doing the same thing over and over again and expecting different results."

By seeing our Frankenstein Monsters through the frank filters of Einstein's teachings, we will notice how much harder it is to continue repressing our laughter as we notice how funny it is when self-proclaimed "intelligent races" of people essentially keep trying to blow each other up in subtle and not so subtle ways. This, despite knowing, as Einstein said, that our separation from "each other" is a kind of "optical illusion of consciousness," in which we are all interconnected within "an illusory albeit very persistent" reality in which duality is a Joke "by which we think and not conditions in which we live." Based on this thinking which is contrary to reality, we keep "doing the same thing over and over again and expecting different results." One can only imagine "God's thoughts" about all these details, and can only suspect that She has a good sense of humor.

The next time a Frankenstein Monster shows up in your life, remember to laugh at how funny it is in light of frank Einstein's teachings.

There is a relativity joke in which Einstein asks the conductor, "Excuse me, does New York stop by this train?"

The real question is: does the station (our Illusory World) we co-created with thought, stop by this train we will co-create with laughter? Will we need to jump on a different train (the "Laughter train") that bypasses our train of thought?

Just before completing this book, I saw a patient who had a health condition. When I told him about a very simple, inexpensive and highly effective treatment for his condition, he behaved as though I was speaking Martian.

It took several hours for the joke to fully hit before realizing that I was doing the same thing regarding a condition I had at the time. Even while writing this book, it took me quite a while to take a dose of the Ho-Ho-Holy medicine and laugh at my own thoughts. But every time I take this medicine, the Jokes become a bit easier to find, and life is more joyful. I hope this book will do the same for you.

Now the choice is yours. As you go out into the great comedy Ashram of life - where hopefully my silly jokes will have been your greatest tragedy, I would like to leave you with three questions:

- Do you want to live in an Illusory World full of chaos and suffering, or do you want to use your suffering as rocket fuel to blast off to the deepest parts of The Zone that are closest to God Consciousness?

- Are you going to put this book on your bookshelf and go back to live as usual in the Illusory World, or are you going to join the "Laughter Movement" and laugh away all your barriers to living in a Heavenly World, and use the infectious power of laughter to help our Global evolution?

- Do you believe the answer to this and every other question will eventually become obvious the more we laugh at the question?

We can't expect to use dualistic thinking to solve the problems it created, especially when it ignores the fundamental laws of physics, because the train we've been riding seems to be on a collision course with reality.

Let's use The Ho-Ho Holiest Medicine to help live the kind of life God intended. Let's have the courage to experience a world beyond our wildest imagination by conveniently Laughing at The Inconvenient Joke.

Being the First to Laugh

If the Joke is so funny, why is no one else laughing?

The obvious answer is that since there is no "other," once we completely laugh at the Joke with each seemingly individualized cell of Our Body (the One Body that makes up Everything in Creation in which everything is Perfectly Interconnected) there is no one else that needs to laugh. We would have laughed our way out of our illusory world, and there would be nothing left at which to laugh.

Another way of looking at this, within the illusion of "other people," is by seeing what happens during a stage hypnosis show. If one person in an audience is hypnotized into clucking like a chicken, it's funny. If more of the audience is hypnotized into clucking like a chicken, it's even funnier. However, if the whole world is hypnotized into clucking like a chicken, it would no longer be funny because there would be no one left outside The Illusion to laugh.

What if the world is like that? What if everyone has been hypnotized into essentially clucking like a chicken, and there's no one left to laugh. Even those outside the hypnotic illusion are afraid to be the first to challenge their cult-ural conditioning?

What if everyone is too chicken to laugh at others clucking like a chicken?

What if the reason mankind is stuck in the Illusory World is that everyone is too chicken to be the first to laugh, believing they would be stoned like the escaping prisoner in Plato's Allegory?

As you may recall, the other prisoners in the cave felt threatened by the one prisoner who broke out of his chains. After seeing a whole new world outside the cave, he came back and told the others what he saw.

But in my allegory, instead of being too chicken about being stoned, we would be excited to be among the few to step outside the Illusory World and come back laughing!

The main difference between a person returning to prisoners with threatening information and a person returning with laughter is that what threatening information can't accomplish, laughter can. Confronting the other prisoners with information that threatens their whole concept of reality can be enormously distressing. But laughter, by bypassing the mind, bypasses objections. This is why comedians can often get away with more pointed social and political criticisms, allowing them to often tell more truths than their journalist counterparts.

Being among the first to laugh at the Inconvenient Joke can be extremely fun and exciting and can bring about the shift our world has been waiting for. Instead of feeling as though we have the monumental task of transforming an overwhelming number of limiting beliefs about how it can be possible to transform Global Chaos into Heaven on Earth through laughter, think of it as having an unlimited supply of excellent fuel for laughter.

Being the first to laugh at the Inconvenient Joke is a bit like Neil Armstrong's first step on the moon. This laughter will be one small giggle for man, one giant belly laugh for mankind.

This belly laugh has the potential to help us become the Neil Armstrongs of our world. It may allow us to explore the Absolute Bliss of our Interconnectedness and dimensions of reality that we can't even imagine through the filters of thoughts.

Accessing altered states of consciousness, whether it is through meditation, deep prayer, deep work on dissolving the smallest distortions on our lens, Divine Belly Laughter, hypnosis, LaughGnosis, or some combination of all the above, can help us know ourselves at the deepest level. This can enable us to experience humanity's true Divine nature of Gnosis in which magic and miracles can happen. This Gnostic State has the potential to help us shift to dimensions of reality far beyond the moon or any other remnants of time and space and make rocket science seem like horse and buggy technology.

But before you allow your imagination to wander too far, there is one not so minor detail to keep in mind. Although much of the information in this book is based on information from the greatest geniuses and Nobel Laureates who ever lived, whether any of this is possible may be completely up to you. After all, this information is based on an illusory book based on an illusory world which you purchased with illusory money.

The only way of knowing whether any of this is possible is by taking the opportunity to explore the Power of Divine Laughter and by deciding for yourself whether it is indeed The Ho-Ho Holiest Medicine.

Out beyond this Illusory World, there is a Heavenly World.
Let's Laugh our way there!

THE END

References

All quotes from A Course in Miracles© are from the First Edition, published in 1975, by the Foundation for Inner Peace, P.O. Box 598, Mill Valley, CA 94942-0598, www.acim.org, and info@acim.org.

Osho quotes reprinted with permission of copyright holder Osho International Foundation, www.osho.com.Source: Be Realistic: Plan For a Miracle.

Chapter 5

1. Pure Consciousness & Non-Duality: Matter, Multiplicity of Forms, Illusion and Light, An Excerpt from the Secret Doctrine Volume IV; July 2018
https://www.researchgate.net/publication/326719333_Pure_Consciousness_Non-Duality_Matter_Multiplicity_of_Forms_Illusion_and_Light_An_Excerpt_from_the_Secret_Doctrine_Volume_IV
2. Holographic Principle and Quantum Physics, Abstract; Zolt´an Batiz, Bhag C. Chauhan; Departmento de Fisica, Instituto Superior T´ecnico; Lisboa-PORTUGAL February 2, 2008; Page 15-16
3. WHAT IS LIFE? The physical aspect of the living cell"-Erwin Schrodinger, 1944
4. As quoted in Schrödinger: Life and Thought (1989) by Walter Moore. Mind and Matter (1958)
5. The David Bohm Society: http://dbohm.com/david-bohm-implicate-order.html
6. Spiritual Science, Eric Dubay, Lulu.com, July 2012
7. Russell Targ, Limitless Mind Pg. 7, New World Library, 2004

Chapter 9

1. Paul Ekman, Goguen-Hughes, Survival of the Kindest. Darwin's belief that altruism is a vital part of life is being confirmed by modern science. Mindful, Taking Time for What Matters, December 23, 2010.
https://www.mindful.org/cooperate/
2. Survival of the Fittest Has Evolved: Try Survival of the Kindest by Christopher Kukk / Mar.08.2017 NBCNews.com
https://www.nbcnews.com/better/relationships/survival-fittest-has-evolved-try-survival-kindest-n730196

Chapter 10

1. First Edition, published in 1975, by the Foundation for Inner Peace, P.O. Box 598, Mill Valley, CA 94942-0598, www.acim.org and info@acim.org, lesson 23

Chapter 13

1. Esther and Jerry Hicks: Ask and It is Given, Learning to Manifest the Law of Attraction, pg. 114 Carlsbad, United States, Hay House, 2008.

2. Dr. David R. Hawkins, MD, Ph.D.: The Map of Consciousness; Power Vs. Force: The Hidden Determinants of Human Behavior. 2002, NewYork. Hay House, Inc.

Chapter 14

1. The hero's Journey started in 1871 with anthropologist Edward Taylor's observations of common patterns in plots of hero's journeys. This version was adapted from the work of Joseph Campbell, Big Picture Questions.com and the work of Trent Thornley.

Chapter 15

1. Samina Salim. Current Neuropharmacol 2014 Mar; 12(2): 140–147

2. Dupond JL1, Humbert P, Taillard C; Relationship between autoimmune diseases and personality traits in women. Presse Med. 1990 Dec 22-29;19(44):2019-22. Article in French
http://www.ncbi.nlm.nih.gov/pubmed/2148613

3. Janice K. Kiecolt-Glaser and Lynanne McGuire; Psychoneuroimmunology: Psychological Influences on Immune Function and Health. Ohio State University College of Medicine. J Consult Clin Psychol. 2002 Jun;70(3):537-47;
http://www.uppitysciencechick.com/kiecolt-glaser_pni_jccp.pdf

4. Kidd PM. Multiple sclerosis, an autoimmune inflammatory disease: prospects for its integrative management. Altern Med Rev. 2001 Dec;6(6):540-66

5. Susan Conova; Is Parkinson's an Autoimmune Disease? Attack by Own Immune System May Kill Neurons in Parkinson's. Columbia University Medical Center Newsroom. April 17, 2014
http://newsroom.cumc.columbia.edu/blog/2014/04/17/parkinsons-autoimmune-disease/

6. D'Andrea MR; Add Alzheimer's disease to the list of autoimmune diseases. Med Hypotheses. 2005;64(3):458-63.
http://www.ncbi.nlm.nih.gov/pubmed/15617848

7. Eskelinen M1, Ollonen P; Assessment of "cancer-prone personality" characteristics in healthy study subjects and in patients with breast disease and breast cancer using the commitment questionnaire: a prospective case-control study in Finland. Anticancer Res. 2011 Nov;31(11):4013-7

8. Kiecolt-Glaser JK1, Glaser R; Psychoneuroimmunology and cancer: fact or fiction? Eur J Cancer. 1999 Oct;35(11):1603-7.
http://www.ncbi.nlm.nih.gov/pubmed/10673969

9. Dr. Bernie Siegel; Prescriptions For Living: Inspirational Lessons for a Joyful, Loving Life, Pg 145-146, Harper Collins Publishers, Inc., 1999

10. Spiegel D, Bloom JR, Kraemer HC, Gottheil E (1989) Effect of psychosocial treatment on survival of patients with metastatic breast cancer. Lancet 2: 888–891
http://www.ncbi.nlm.nih.gov/pubmed/2571815

11. Arthroscopic debridement for osteoarthritis of the knee. Cochrane Database of Systematic Reviews: This version published: 2008; Review content assessed as up-to-date: November 11, 2007.
http://www.ncbi.nlm.nih.gov/pubmedhealth/PMH0013262/

12. http://learn.genetics.utah.edu/content/epigenetics/twins/

13. Susan Krauss Whitbourne Ph.D.; Can you survive your personality? Psychology Today;
https://www.psychologytoday.com/blog/fulfillment-any-age/201009/can-you-survive-your-personality

14. Spiegel D, Bloom JR. Patients with metastatic breast cancer benefited from self-hypnosis and from participation in group support. Despite a lack of specific suggestions, the women benefited with significantly less pain and an increased duration of survival. Group therapy and hypnosis reduce metastatic breast carcinoma pain. Psychosom Med. 1983;45:333-339

15. Spiegel D, Bloom JR, Kraemer HC, Gottheil E. Effect of psychosocial treatment on survival of patients with metastatic breast cancer. Lancet. 1989; 2:888-891

16. Clawson TA Jr, Swade RH; An untapped potential for hypnosis for cancer treatment is the reported ability to alter regional blood flow, which offers the prospect of increasing the delivery of chemotherapy to a tumour or reducing blood flow to it. The hypnotic control of blood flow and pain: the cure of warts and the potential for the use of hypnosis in the treatment of cancer. Am J Clin Hypn. 1975;17:160-169

Chapter 16

1. Visual function in multiple personality disorder. J Am Optom Assoc. Birnbaum M, Thomann K. 1996 Jun;67(6):327-34.
http://www.ncbi.nlm.nih.gov/pubmed/8888853

2. M. Talbot; Holographic Universe, pg. 99
http://archive.org/stream/HolographicModelOfTheUniverse/holouni_djvu.txt

3. https://www.nytimes.com/1988/06/28/science/probing-the-enigma-of-multiple-personality.html
Probing the Enigma of Multiple Personality. By Daniel Goleman June 28, 1988

4. Daniel Goleman, "New Focus on Multiple Personality " New York Times. May 21, 1985

5. Robert Phillips, Jr., a psychologist reported that tumors can appear and disappear Truddi Chase, When Rabbit Howls (New York: E. P. Dutton, 1987). Taken from:
http://archive.org/stream/HolographicModelOfTheUniverse/holouni_djvu.txt

6. Rossi, Ernest and Cheek, David. Mind-Body Therapy: Methods of Ideodynamic Healing in Hypnosis. W.W Norton & Co. New York and London, 1988 pg. 183

7. Hudson, T (1893). The law of Psychic phenomena. Chicago: A.C. McClurg.

8. Eliott C. McLaughlin; "Dead Mississippi man begins breathing in embalming room, coroner says" CNN. March 2, 2014,

http://edition.cnn.com/2014/02/28/us/dead-man-comes-back-life/

Chapter 19

1. Laughter Wellness Benefits: http://www.invokelaughter.com/benefits2/

2. Want to Live Longer? Carry on Laughing; Tuesday 16 December 2008; Independent Digital News & Media, London, U.K.

3. "Laugh Lots, Live Longer" Scientific American, By Tori Rodriguez on September 1, 2016

https://www.scientificamerican.com/article/laugh-lots-live-longer/

4. Smile Intensity in Photographs Predicts Longevity; Ernest L. Abel, Michael L. Kruger First Published February 26, 2010

https://journals.sagepub.com/doi/abs/10.1177/0956797610363775?journalCode=pssa

5. The Untapped Power Of Smiling; Forbes Magazine, Mar 22, 2011; Eric Savitz; Guest Post Written by Ron Gutman

Chapter 22

1. Robert Preidt Health Day Reporter; SUNDAY, April 27, 2014 (HealthDay News); Published on Web MD on the internet

http://www.webmd.com/mental-health/news/20140427/laughter-may-work-like-meditation-in-the-brain

2. http://web.stanford.edu/group/hopes/cgi-bin/hopes_test/meditation-and-hd/

3. Understanding Your Brain, Jeffrey L. Fannin, Ph.D.

http://drjoedispenza.com/files/understanding-brainwaves_white_paper.pdf

4. http://www.explorations-in-consciousness.com/forums/index.php?threads/gamma-oscillations.3842/

Chapter 23

1. http://www.integrativepainmd.com/hypnosis/

Made in the USA
Monee, IL
14 June 2020